# Lethal Diseases of the Ascending Aorta

Proceedings of the Symposium *Frontiers of Medicine,*
held at The University of Chicago, Chicago, Illinois
December 18, 1974

# Lethal Diseases of the Ascending Aorta

Edited by
Constantine E. Anagnostopoulos, M.D., D.Sc.

Associate Professor of Surgery
Senior Cardiac Surgeon
The University of Chicago

University Park Press
Baltimore · London · Tokyo

**UNIVERSITY PARK PRESS**
International Publishers in Science and Medicine
Chamber of Commerce Building
Baltimore, Maryland 21202



Typeset by The Composing Room of Michigan, Inc.

Manufactured in the United States of America by Universal Lithographers, Inc., and The Maple Press Co., Inc.



**Library of Congress Cataloging in Publication Data**

Symposium Frontiers of Medicine, University of Chicago, 1974.
Lethal diseases of the ascending aorta.

Includes index.
1. Aorta—Diseases—Congresses. 2. Coronary heart disease—Congresses. 3. Aorta—Surgery—Congresses. I. Anagnostopoulos, Constantine E., 1940- II. Title. [DNLM: 1. Aortic diseases—Congresses. WG410 S989L 1974]
RC691.S94 1974 616.1'38 75-35781
ISBN 0-8391-0889-3

# Contents

Contributors vii
Welcome ix
*D. B. Skinner*
Preface xi
*C. E. Anagnostopoulos*
Acknowledgments xii
*C. E. Anagnostopoulos*
Dedication xiii

**I. CORONARY DISEASE**

1. Severe Stenosis of the Left Main Coronary Artery
*D. C. Sabiston, Jr.* 2
2. Pre-Infarction Angina in Left Main Coronary Artery Disease
*P. J. Scanlon, J. V. Talano, R. Nemickas, R. Pifarre, J. M. Moran, and R. M. Gunnar* 18
3. Angiographic Diagnosis of Left Main Coronary Artery Disease
*R. E. Falicov* 27
4. Unstable Angina Pectoris
*L. Resnekov, J. Al-Sadir, R. E. Falicov, and C. E. Anagnostopoulos* 37
5. Panel on Coronary Disease
Moderator: *L. Resnekov*
Panel Members: *R. M. Gunnar, R. E. Falicov, J. M. Moran, J. J. Lamberti, and C. E. Anagnostopoulos* 49

**II. TRANSPOSITION**

6. Complete Transposition of the Great Arteries: Physiology, Diagnosis, and Medical Management
*R. A. Arcilla* 54
7. Surgical Treatment of Transposition of the Great Arteries: Technical Considerations and Results
*D. A. Cooley* 77
8. Panel on Transposition
Moderator: *R. L. Replogle*
Panel Members: *D. A. Cooley, R. A. Arcilla, N. E. Shumway, and C. E. Anagnostopoulos* 92

**III. DISSECTIONS**

9. Acute Aortic Dissections: Introduction and Medical Therapy
*C. L. Athanasuleas, C. E. Anagnostopoulos, and L. Resnekov* 98

10. The Aorta in the Marfan Syndrome and Other Genetic Disorders of Connective Tissue
*V. A. McKusick* 113
11. Surgical Therapy of Dissection of the Aorta
*N. E. Shumway and R. B. Griepp* 124
12. Cardiac Anesthesia for Lethal Diseases of the Ascending Aorta
*C.-Y. Lin and D. W. Benson* 129
13. Panel on Acute Aortic Dissection
Moderator: *D. A. Cooley*
Panel Members: *V. A. McKusick, N. E. Shumway, and C. E. Anagnostopoulos* 144

Index 149

# Contributors

**Jafar Al-Sadir, M.D.**
Assistant Professor of Medicine (Cardiology), The University of Chicago

**C. E. Anagnostopoulos, M.D., D.Sc.**
Associate Professor of Surgery, Senior Cardiac Surgeon, The University of Chicago

**Rene A. Arcilla, M.D.**
Professor of Pediatrics, Chief of Pediatric Cardiology, The University of Chicago

**Constantine L. Athanasuleas, M.D.**
Pritzker School of Medicine, The University of Chicago

**Donald W. Benson, M.D.**
Professor and Chairman, Department of Anesthesiology, The University of Chicago

**Denton A. Cooley, M.D.**
Surgeon-in-Chief, Texas Heart Institute

**Raul E. Falicov, M.D.**
Associate Professor of Medicine, Director of Clinical Hemodynamics, The University of Chicago

**Randall B. Griepp, M.D.**
Assistant Professor of Cardiac Surgery, Stanford University

**Rolf M. Gunnar, M.D.**
Chief, Section of Cardiology, Professor of Medicine, Loyola University

**John J. Lamberti, M.D.**
Assistant Professor of Surgery (Thoracic and Cardiovascular), The University of Chicago

**Chung-Yuan Lin, M.D.**
Associate Professor of Anesthesiology, Chief of Cardiac Anesthesia, The University of Chicago

**Victor A. McKusick, M.D.**
Professor and Chairman Department of Medicine, Johns Hopkins University

**John M. Moran, M.D.**
Associate Professor of Surgery, (Thoracic and Cardiovascular Section), Loyola University

**Rimgaudas Nemickas, M.D.**
Associate Chief, Section of Cardiology and Director of Cardiac Care Unit, Associate Professor of Medicine, Loyola University

**Roque Pifarre, M.D.**
Chief, Cardiopulmonary Surgery Section, Professor of Surgery, Loyola University

**Robert L. Replogle, M.D.**
Professor of Surgery, Chief of Cardiac Surgery, The University of Chicago

**Leon Resnekov, M.D.**
Professor of Medicine,
Joint Chief, Cardiology,
The University of Chicago

**David C. Sabiston, Jr., M.D.**
James P. Duke Professor and Chairman Department of Surgery, Duke University

**P. J. Scanlon, M.D.**
Director, Cardiopulmonary Laboratory and Associate Professor of Medicine, Loyola University

**Norman E. Shumway, M.D.**
Professor and Chairman of Cardiac Surgery, Stanford University

**David B. Skinner, M.D.**
Dallas B. Phemister Professor and Chairman Department of Surgery, The University of Chicago

**James V. Talano, M.D.**
Assistant Professor of Medicine, Loyola University

# Welcome

Welcome to a very special edition of The Frontiers of Medicine. I shall take a few minutes to tell you what has been going on in the cardiovascular disease field at The University of Chicago in the past couple of years.

A little over two years ago President Levi, the Trustees, the Central Administration, and Deans made a commitment to strengthening both clinical and research activities in cardiovascular disease. Since that time a great deal has happened. We established a separate cardiac surgery service and restructured the entire faculty in this field. Dr. Robert Replogle has been appointed chief of the cardiac surgery service and promoted to professor. Dr. Anagnostopoulos has been appointed as the senior attending cardiac surgeon and promoted to associate professor. And we have added two new faculty members in Cardiac Surgery: Dr. John Lamberti from the Peter Bent Brigham Hospital and the Boston Children's Hospital, and Dr. Tom DeMeester from Johns Hopkins by way of the U.S. Army.

In the meantime the Cardiology section has remained as strong as it always has been under the leadership of Drs. Fozzard and Resnekov as joint-chiefs of adult cardiology. The diagnostic laboratories have been assigned to Drs. Falicov and Brooks and their hemodynamic studies have become an outstanding part of our program. In addition, four new faculty members have been added to the cardiology section this year: Drs. Arnsdorf, Ford, Romero, and DasGupta. They each have strong clinical interests and have helped us a great deal in our clinic and cardiology program.

In Pediatric Cardiology, Drs. Arcilla, Thilenius, and colleagues have maintained and strengthened their international reputation in a very active children's heart surgery program.

In other areas we have made significant changes. In Anesthesiology we have created a section of cardiovascular anesthesia headed by Dr. Chung Lin, cardiac surgeon and anesthesiologist. Dr. Donald Benson joins us as Chairman of the Department of Anesthesiology, having served for the last 18 years as Chief of Anesthesiology at Johns Hopkins.

In Radiology significant changes have been occurring. The appointment of Dr. John Fennessey as the new Chairman of the Department of Radiology brings a distinguished chest diagnostician into the leadership of that department, and he is taking efforts to upgrade our resources in cardiovascular radiology. The first important step was the return of Dr. C. T. Lu to our faculty as a full-time member. Dr. Lu is an expert in angiographic technique and together with Dr. Collins adds to our resources. In the research area Dr. Paul Harper's work on myocardial scanning aids our understanding of ischemic heart disease.

Dr. Seymour Glagov has become the Chief of a Cardiovascular Pathology program and has collaborated with many of us in clinical and research projects.

We have created a new section of clinical pharmacology which will be headed by Dr. Leon Goldberg, formerly of Emory University. One of his major interests is cardiovascular drugs.

Our traditional strength in basic science and research continues with the research activities of Drs. Rabinowitz, Page, and Fischman in muscle disorders. Drs. Robbins and Scanu are involved in studies of protein coagulation and Dr. Wissler continues to apply himself to the problem of atherosclerosis and its possible prevention or cure.

Our faculty now is strong in the cardiovascular sciences. We believe there has been a significant development of the program with a new strength and hence a reason for celebration. In addition we have upgraded our facilities during the past two years; a new Hans Hecht Cardiovascular Diagnostic Laboratory was opened this past month. This is dedicated to Dr. Hecht, former Chief of Cardiology and Chairman of Medicine here. It gives us a modern facility for diagnostic catheterization and angiography studies. The laboratory will be directed by Drs. Falicov and Brooks.

You probably have seen a large hole in the ground in front of this building. This is the site for a new surgery and brain research institute. Included within the six-story building will be new facilities for cardiovascular surgery and research.

The Pediatric Cardiac Catheterization Laboratory directed by Drs. Arcilla and Thilenius has been remodeled recently. Our facilities now match the capabilities of our faculty.

Our program in research remains strong. In addition to the NIH-funded Special Center for atherosclerosis research headed by Dr. Wissler, within the last 12 months we were designated as a Special Center by the NIH for research into ischemic heart disease headed by Dr. Resnekov; this is a multidisciplinary program and involves many of the faculty.

We have now assembled the faculty, have built or are building facilities, have developed programs, and are clearly attracting new patients to accomplish the objective of the University Administration when they decided to help us strengthen our program in cardiovascular disease. As our celebration we have gathered distinguished visiting faculty in a discussion of lethal diseases of the aorta which remain among the most challenging and difficult in their diagnostic, therapeutic, and etiological aspects.

I introduce Dr. Anagnostopoulos. He is our Senior Cardiac Surgeon and Associate Professor of Surgery and has done the difficult leg work in organizing this program.

David B. Skinner

# Preface

The present monograph represents the proceedings of the December 18, 1974 Frontiers of Medicine Symposium held at The University of Chicago on the topic of Lethal Diseases of the Ascending Aorta.

The clinical presentation, diagnostic and therapeutic aspects of these life-threatening, frequently neglected diseases of the ascending aorta and coronary arteries are the subjects of this conference. The diseases are all common. Transposition is the most common cause of death from congenital heart disease in the first year of life. Acute dissection is the most common catastrophe involving the human aorta. And main left coronary obstruction is a frequent cause of unstable angina. In addition to sharing anatomic proximity, these formerly incurable emergencies are now palliated successfully by means of surgery.

C. E. Anagnostopoulos

# Acknowledgments

The editor would like to thank Dr. Louis Cohen, Professor of Medicine (Cardiology), The University of Chicago, for his encouragement and support of this conference which was held as part of the Frontiers of Medicine Series. In addition, thanks are due to the E. F. Andrews Foundation, Chicago, Illinois, and the Combined Cardiac Research Fund of the Department of Surgery, The University of Chicago, supported by generous donations of friends and patients in our Combined Cardiac Service.

The publication of this monograph was made possible by the untiring efforts of my secretary, Mrs. Marilyn Zarowny, and Mr. Joseph Kozicki, Manager, Biological Sciences Division, Audio-Visual Department, The University of Chicago.

Finally, the editor is grateful to Mr. Paul Brookes and Ms. Betsy Webb of University Park Press for their extraordinary cooperation and patience in the preparation and prompt completion of this book.

C. E. Anagnostopoulos

*to our patients*

# Coronary Disease

# I

Severe Stenosis of the Left Main Coronary Artery

Pre-Infarction Angina in Left Main Coronary Artery Disease

Angiographic Diagnosis of Left Main Coronary Artery Disease

Unstable Angina Pectoris

Panel on Coronary Disease

# 1 Severe Stenosis of the Left Main Coronary Artery

D. C. Sabiston, Jr., M.D.

In the recent past increased recognition has been given the fact that severe stenosis of the left main coronary artery represents a critical disorder associated with a poor prognosis. In 1972, Cohen and associates, among others, directed attention to the high mortality associated with this lesion if untreated, 50% in a 2-year period after diagnosis by arteriography (1). Lavine and associates (2) reported 30 patients with left main coronary arterial lesions, and among those in whom operation was not performed, the mortality was 33%, all deaths occurring within 1 month after arteriography. In a further study, a 5-year mortality from the time of arteriographic recognition of critical stenosis of the left main coronary artery was 57% (3). It is now clear that such patients are characterized by a high risk, and recent data indicate that survival is clearly improved in those patients managed by early operation.

## ANATOMY OF THE LEFT MAIN CORONARY ARTERY

The left coronary artery arises from the left coronary sinus and its length is usually 10 mm. but is not infrequently shorter. However, the length may vary from 2 to 3 mm. to as much as 40 mm. before bifurcation into the left anterior descending and left circumflex branches (4). Rarely, there is no left main coronary but rather the left circumflex and anterior descending coronary arteries arise from separate orifices of the left sinus of Valsalva.

## PATHOLOGICAL MANIFESTATIONS

In most reports in which the left main coronary artery (LCA) has a stenosis of 70% or more, there is a high incidence of involvement of the other coronary arteries. In Zeft's series of 56 patients with left main coronary stenosis of at least 75%, in half the lesion was 90% or more (5), 34 had 75% or greater stenosis of the left anterior descending (LAD), and 32 had a similar lesion in the circumflex (CF). Of the 56 patients, 26 had severe associated disease of *both* the anterior descending and circumflex branches. In addition, 37 patients had a 75% or greater lesion in the right coronary artery (RC). Of considerable interest is the fact that only *three* of these 56 patients (8%) had isolated disease of the left main coronary.

In a study by Khaja of 28 patients (6), 22 had a 75 to 90% lesion in the LCA and three had a 50 to 75% lesion. In three patients, the arteriograms demonstrated a *total* occlusion of the LCA. Associated lesions, with more than 50% narrowing, were found in the LAD in 22 patients, in the CF or its marginal branches in 18 patients, and in the right coronary in 23 patients.

In a series of 30 patients studied by Lavine and associates (2), 29 had two or three vessel disease. Significant coronary arterial collateral vessels were noted in 21 patients. In our own series at Duke, Kisslo and associates (7) recently studied 1003 patients with complete right and left cardiac catheterization, cardiac output, left ventriculography, and coronary arteriography. In this group of 1003 patients, 101 (10.1%) had 70% or more stenotic lesion in the LCA. In addition, 104 (10.4%) had a definite LCA lesion, but it was less than 70%. In the remaining 798 patients (79.5%), the LCA was normal. The prevalence of associated triple vessel disease was impressive, with 70% or greater narrowing of the anterior descending in 68 of the 101 patients (67%). In this series, *six* patients had isolated disease of the left main coronary artery without evidence of significant arterial disease elsewhere. Of particular interest were four patients who had *total occlusion* of the left main coronary artery.

## CLINICAL MANIFESTATIONS

An increasing prevalence of severe left main coronary disease is generally noted with increasing age and in the Duke series of 101 patients with severe stenosis of the LCA, it is interesting that more than 20% of the patients were over 60 years of age (7). Other clinical features include a higher incidence of classical angina (80% or more). It has also been shown that clinical recognition of patients with severe narrowing of the left main coronary artery may be based on the results of graded exercise tolerance testing (1, 2). In studies from our own laboratory by Bartel and associates (8), patients with LCA lesions were more often found to manifest profound S-T segment changes during exercise compared with those in whom the branches were involved.

Mortality from aorto-coronary saphenous vein bypass grafts in patients with significant LCA lesions was reported by Pichard at 8.1% (9), by Lavine at 11% (2), by Zeft at 10.7% (5), and by Khaja at 28% (6). In our own experience since 1973 of 22 patients, there were three deaths (14%).

Emphasis has also been placed by several authors not only on the natural history of the disease but also on the risk of coronary arteriography. For example, Lavine reported that among 30 patients with LCA lesions undergoing coronary arteriography there were three deaths (10%). In the Duke series, there has been only one death in patients with significant LCA disease at the time of arteriography among the 101 studied (1%).

Several authors have reported that left coronary artery stenosis is generally associated with an older patient population, with a more classic history of angina pectoris than that of coronary artery disease at large, and with frequent calcification being seen in the area of the left coronary artery. Moreover, the electrocardiographic findings following exercise are apt to be more strongly positive. Most patients in this group show 2 mm. or more of S-T depression during exercise testing. Khaja's group showed a graft patency of 84% (6). They also showed a 77% S-T depression of 2 mm. or more, and Cohen's series showed this figure to be 82% (1). An abnormal ventriculogram was present in 60% of Khaja's study (6), 70% of Cohen's study (1), and 86% in Lavine's study (2). In addition, multiple vessel disease is quite common. Emphasis has also been placed upon the fact that, during the initiation of anesthesia preparatory to surgery, serious arrhythmias and hypotension are more apt to occur in this group. *Unstable angina* is common and in some series has been unusually high. For example, in the series of Zeft it was 75% (5).

## SURGICAL RESULTS

Symptomatic improvement is the rule following operation. Zeft reported 90% of those surviving operation had significant reduction in anginal pain and 76% were totally asymptomatic. Postoperative catheterization showed a patency rate of 83% (5). In Lavine's series of 16 survivors following operation, all were clinically improved (2). Symptomatic improvement was substantiated by normalization or improved response to exercise testing in seven of eight patients studied 6 months following operation (6).

## DISCUSSION

Within the past several years, it has become increasingly apparent that significant stenosis of the left main coronary artery is a very serious lesion and is probably the most ominous single atherosclerotic lesion involving the coronary circulation. The high mortality associated with the natural history of the disease as well as the increased surgical risk as compared with patients with other types of coronary obstruction are also significant. In a recent report from the University of Michigan, it was shown that, among 17 patients with a left main coronary lesion greater than 50%, eight died within 1 to 23 months after arteriography (10). It has become apparent that several distinct features help to characterize the clinical syndrome. These include its presence in a somewhat older group, the fact that classical angina is present with a higher frequency, and that calcification of the left main coronary artery is often observed. In addition, it has been noted that the exercise stress test shows a higher incidence of a 2-mm. or greater S-T depression in this group.

It has become quite clear that patients with critical lesions in the left main coronary artery in whom symptoms of pre-infarction angina are present represent a surgical emergency and should be operated on without delay. In a consideration of this problem, it is of interest to reflect upon the fact that the first proven case of premortem diagnosis of acute myocardial infarction by Herrick in 1912 was made in a patient with a severe lesion of the left main coronary artery (Fig. 1) (11). To quote Herrick directly:

> "A man, aged 55, supposedly in good health, was seized an hour after a moderately full meal with severe pain in the lower precordial region. He was nauseated and, believing that something he had just eaten had disagreed with him, he induced vomiting by tickling his throat. The pain continued, however, and his physician was called, who found him cold, nauseated, with small rapid pulse, and suffering extreme pain. The stomach was washed out and morphine given hypodermically. The pain did not cease *until three hours had passed.*[1] From this time the patient remained in bed, free from pain, but the pulse continued rapid and small, and numerous rales appeared in the chest, When I saw him twelve hours from the painful attack his mind was clear and calm. The chest was full of fine and coarse moist rales; there was a running, feeble pulse of 140. The heart tones were very faint and there was a most startling and confusing hyperresonance over the chest, the area of

[1] Italics added for emphasis of duration of pain.

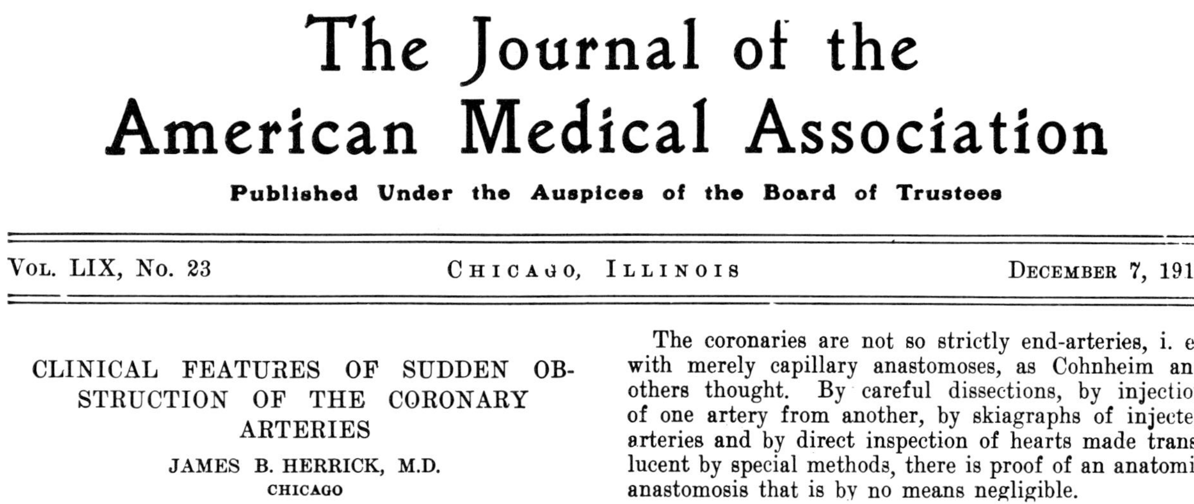

# The Journal of the American Medical Association

Published Under the Auspices of the Board of Trustees

VOL. LIX, NO. 23 — CHICAGO, ILLINOIS — DECEMBER 7, 1912

## CLINICAL FEATURES OF SUDDEN OBSTRUCTION OF THE CORONARY ARTERIES

JAMES B. HERRICK, M.D.
CHICAGO

The coronaries are not so strictly end-arteries, i. e., with merely capillary anastomoses, as Cohnheim and others thought. By careful dissections, by injection of one artery from another, by skiagraphs of injected arteries and by direct inspection of hearts made translucent by special methods, there is proof of an anatomic anastomosis that is by no means negligible.

Figure 1. Title page of Herrick's classical paper which represents the first premortem diagnosis of acute myocardial infarction.

heart dullness being entirely obscured. The abdomen was tympanitic. The urine was scanty, of high specific gravity, and contained a small amount of albumin and a few casts. The temperature was subnormal, later going to 99° F. Occasionally there was nausea and twice a sudden projectile vomiting of considerable fluid material. This condition remained with slight variations up to the time of death, fifty-two hours after the onset of pain, though at one time the rales seemed nearly to have disappeared. A few hours before death the patient described a slight pain in the heart region, but said it did not amount to much. A remarkable circumstance, and one that occasioned surprise in those who saw the patient and who realized from the almost imperceptible pulse and the feeble heart tones how weak the heart must be, was the fact that he frequently indulged in active muscular effort without evident harm. He rolled vigorously from side to side in the bed, sat suddenly bolt upright, or reached out to take things from the table near by; and once, feeling a sudden nausea, he jumped out of bed, dodged the nurse and ran into the bathroom, where he vomited; and yet he seemed none the worse for these exertions.

*Necropsy* (Dr. Hektoen). The heart was of normal size, but both coronary arteries were markedly sclerotic, with calcareous districts and narrowing of the lumen. A short distance from its origin the left coronary artery was completely obliterated by a red thrombus that had formed *at a point of great narrowing.*[2] The wall of the left ventricle showed well-marked areas of yellowish and reddish softening, especially extensive in the interventricular septum. At the very apex the muscle was decidedly softer than elsewhere. The beginning of the aorta showed a few yellowish spots, these areas becoming less marked as the descending part was reached. An acute fibrinous pericardial deposit, which showed no bacteria in smears, was found over the left ventricle. (The pericarditis probably explains the slighter pain complained of a few hours before death.) There was marked edema of the lungs. In other respects the anatomic findings were those of health."

In this classic paper, Herrick also mentioned that a colleague had related to him the case of a man, aged 60 years, who 3 days after a severe anginal seizure felt well enough to walk on the street, but with some dyspnea. He died *suddenly* on the 5th day and at autopsy, obstruction in the left coronary was found similar to that in the patient Herrick himself has reported.

It is also interesting that Herrick was aware of Fraentzel's instructive case of Professor Panum (12). Herrick reported that for a few weeks Panum had noticed dyspnea and a tight feeling upon climbing stairs. In 1885, upon walking home in the wind, he was forced to stop frequently and when he reached home had a sudden severe, tearing pain in the precordium, which extended to the left arm and fingers. His pulse became rapid, small, and irregular and he broke out into a profuse sweat. He was nauseated but his mind was apparently quite clear. Some 14 hours later he

[2] Italics added.

died suddenly and at autopsy, the left coronary artery was markedly atheromatous and narrowed with a white thrombus attached to its wall. Moreover, there was a rupture of the left ventricle. It is rather remarkable today to reflect upon these superbly described *early* reports of lesions of the left main coronary artery and to recognize that in the recent past the severity of this condition has been re-emphasized.

It is perhaps worthy to recall again the classic description of Heberden in 1759 of the clinical manifestations of angina pectoris, observations made long before there was any known association between this symptom complex and disease of the heart (13). Heberden said:

> "There is a disorder of the chest marked with strong and peculiar symptoms, considerable for the kind of danger belonging to it, and not extremely rare, which deserves to be mentioned more at length. The seat of it, and sense of strangling, and anxiety with which it is attended may make it not improperly be called *angina pectoris.*[3]
>
> They who are afflicted with it, are seized while they are walking (more especially if it be up hill, and soon after eating) with a painful and most disagreeable sensation in the chest, which seems as if it would extinguish life, if it were to increase or continue; but the moment they stand still, all this uneasiness vanishes.
>
> In all other respects, the patients are, at the beginning of the disorder, perfectly well, and in particular have no shortness of breath from which it is totally different. The pain is sometimes situated in the upper part, sometimes in the middle, sometimes at the bottom of the sternum, and often more inclined to the left than to the right. It likewise very frequently extends from the chest to the middle of the left arm. The pulse is, at least sometimes, not disturbed by this pain, as I have had opportunities of observing by feeling the pulse during the paroxysm. Males are most liable to that disease, especially such as have passed their fiftieth year.
>
> After it has continued a year or more, it will not cease so instantaneously upon standing still; and it will come on not only when the persons are walking, but when they are lying down, especially if they lie on their left side, and oblige them to rise up out of their beds. In some inveterate cases it has been brought on by the motion of a horse, or a carriage, and even by swallowing, coughing, going to stool, or speaking, or any disturbance of the mind. . . .
>
> The termination of the angina pectoris is remarkable. For, if no accidents intervene, but the disease go on to its height, the patients all suddenly fall down, and perish almost immediately. Of which indeed their frequent faintness, and sensations as if all the powers of life were failing, afford no obscure intimation."

However, the possibility of an association between anginal symptoms and coronary disease began to be suspected and by 1897, Osler was to say in his magnificent treatise entitled "Lectures on Angina Pectoris and Allied

[3] Italics added.

States" the following: "It is easy to suppose that a narrowing of the orifices of the coronary arteries, or of the lumen of a main branch, can bring about conditions most favorable for the production of this intermittent claudication–i.e., a state in which, so long as the heart is acting quietly, sufficient blood reaches its muscle; but if called upon to act more forcibly, by exertion or emotion, the larger supply, then needful to maintain the nutrition, might not be forthcoming, with the result of a relative ischemia and disturbance of function. What is the condition of the heart muscle in this ischemia? Is it likely to be the same in the narrowing of atheroma and in the blocking from thrombosis and embolism?" (14) One must admire Osler's brilliance and clear ability to correlate clinical and pathological findings as evidenced by this classic statement.

The beginning of the author's experience with severe stenosis of the left main coronary artery began in 1964 when asked to see a 39-year-old patient with severe angina pectoris. At the time of coronary arteriography, the tip of the catheter could not be made to enter the left coronary orifice because of the marked stenosis. Therefore, dye was injected into the left sinus of Valsalva, which demonstrated an almost totally occluded left main coronary artery with post-stenotic dilatation (Fig. 2) (15). Much thought was given to the most appropriate means of surgical treatment of this condition. Two years earlier, on April 4, 1962, a patient with a completely occluded right coronary artery had been treated by an anastomosis of a saphenous vein graft from the side of the ascending aorta to the end of the right coronary artery, as shown in Figure 3 (15). An illustration of this operation was made at the time by the well-known medical artist, Leon Schlossberg. The procedure was performed with the use of a partially occluding clamp placed on the aorta for the proximal anastomosis. This allowed the heart to maintain the cardiac output and extracorporeal circulation was not employed. The distal end of the saphenous vein graft was anastomosed to the right coronary artery distal to the total obstruction. Initially, we were quite pleased with the results in this patient and felt that the technique might offer much in the future management of these lesions. However, we were subsequently discouraged in the postoperative period since the patient sustained a cerebrovascular accident and later died. At postmortem examination, a thrombus was demonstrated at the aortic end of the coronary artery anastomosis and it was felt that an embolus from this site could have produced the patient's cerebrovascular accident and we were fearful to employ it again. Therefore, in attacking these severe left main coronary artery lesions, the ascending aorta was opened with excision of a portion of the intra-arterial obstruction of the left coronary artery from within the aorta and also combining it with an incision in the artery itself with removal of additional occluding material

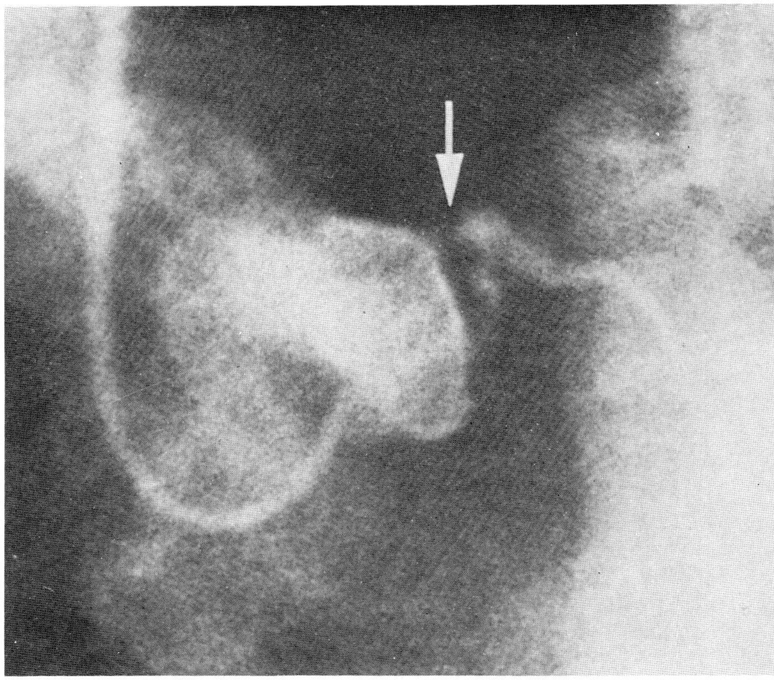

Figure 2. Preoperative arteriogram showing severe stenosis of the left main coronary artery in a 39-year-old patient in 1964. (From Sabiston, D. C., Jr. 1974. The coronary circulation. The William F. Rienhoff, Jr. Lecture. The Johns Hopkins Medical Journal, 134: 314.)

and the placement of a pericardial patch graft to enlarge the area as shown in Figure 4 (15). During this procedure, the left coronary artery and its anterior descending and circumflex branches were continuously perfused with oxygenated blood as illustrated in Figure 4 (15). Fortunately, the patient made an uneventful recovery. A postoperative arteriogram performed at 5 months showed excellent filling of both the left main coronary artery and its branches (Fig. 5) (15). The patient has remained asymptomatic now for nearly 11 years and at present works daily.

The management of severe stenotic lesions of the left main coronary artery is now generally agreed to be bypass graft surgery. It is interesting to reflect upon our surgical heritage in the evolution of this procedure. The first successful use of vein graft to be interposed in the arterial system was performed by Goyanes in Spain in 1906 (16). He reported a patient with a popliteal aneurysm in whom a segment of popliteal vein was excised and utilized as a graft joining the two ends of the proximal and distal

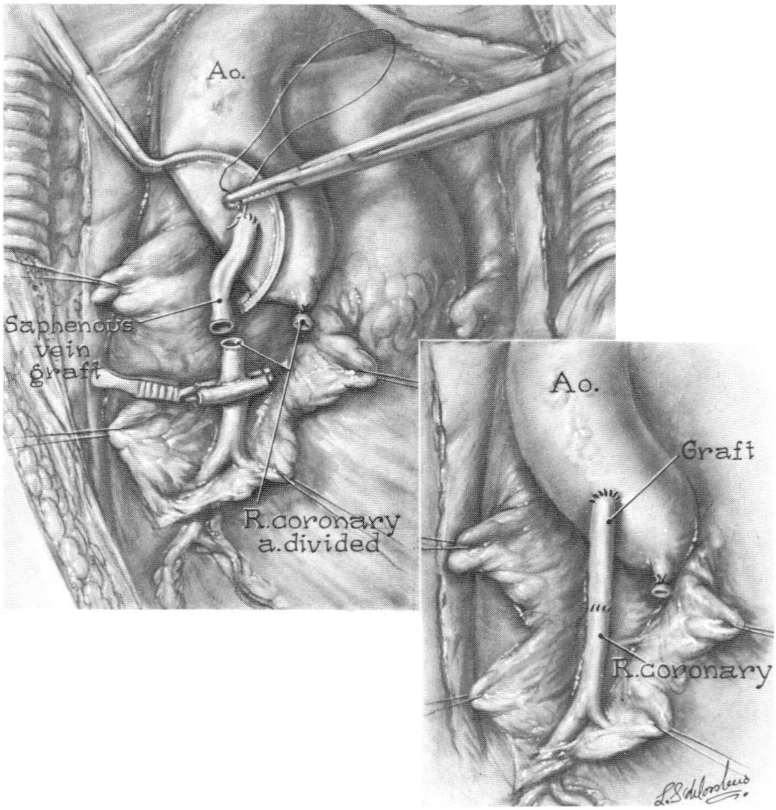


Figure 3. Illustration of use of saphenous vein autograft anastomosed from the ascending aorta to the right coronary artery for proximal coronary arterial occlusion. (From Sabiston, D. C., Jr. 1974. The coronary circulation. The William F. Rienhoff, Jr. Lecture. The Johns Hopkins Medical Journal, 134: 314.)

artery. Following this, Professor Erich Lexer of Konigsberg reported a patient with a large false aneurysm in the axilla secondary to subcoracoid dislocation of the shoulder managed by a vein graft (17). He had also previously used a venous graft in the management of a popliteal aneurysm and the graft functioned well, but the patient died on the 5th postoperative day of delirium tremens. In the United States, Bernheim was the first to employ successfully a vein graft in a patient with a popliteal aneurysm in 1915 (Figs. 6–9) (18).

The use of venous autografts in the coronary circulation was suggested experimentally by Gordon Murray and early observations in the laboratory were published in 1954 (19). In 1962, the author used a saphenous vein

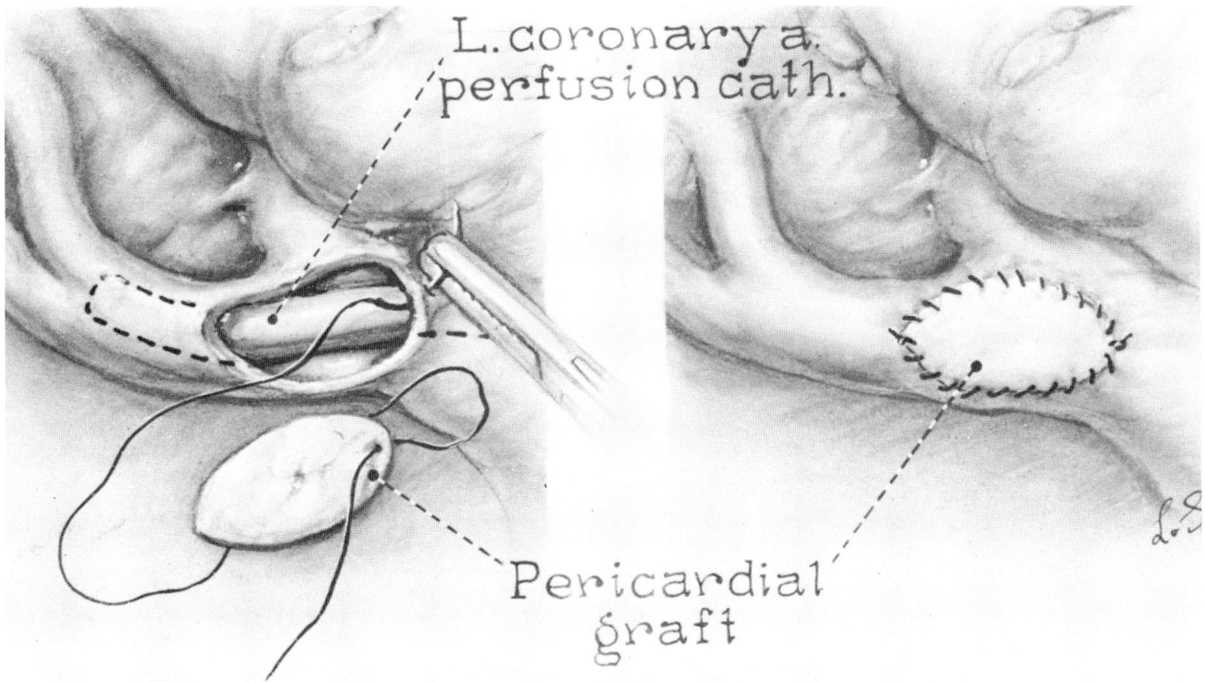


Figure 4. Operative correction of a severe left main coronary arterial lesion shown in arteriogram in Figure 2. See text for description of surgical details. (From Sabiston, D. C., Jr. 1974. The coronary circulation. The William F. Rienhoff, Jr. Lecture. The Johns Hopkins Medical Journal, 134: 314.)

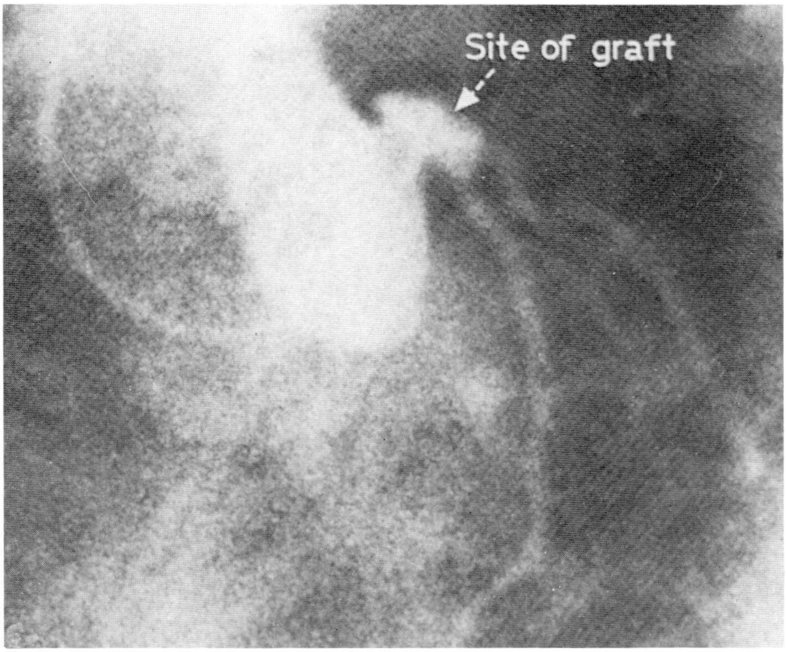


Figure 5. Postoperative arteriogram obtained 5 months after surgical correction of severe left main coronary arterial lesion. The patient remains asymptomatic 10 years after surgical correction. (From Sabiston, D. C., Jr. 1974. The coronary circulation. The William F. Rienhoff, Jr. Lecture. The Johns Hopkins Medical Journal, 134: 314.)

autograft to replace a stenosis of the proximal portion of the right coronary artery (15), but the patient subsequently died after a cerebrovascular accident. In 1964, Garrett and associates used a saphenous vein autograft for the surgical correction of a lesion in the left main coronary and later reported a 7-year follow-up with patency (20). Much credit is due Favaloro (21) and Johnson (22) for their pioneering contributions in popularizing the use of saphenous vein autografts in the surgical management of patients with occluding coronary lesions. Since that time, thousands of patients with severe angina pectoris have been relieved by this procedure and it is currently the most frequently performed operation in cardiac surgery.

## SUMMARY

Severe stenosis of the left main coronary artery has been recognized in the recent past to be associated with a very poor prognosis. The lesion is

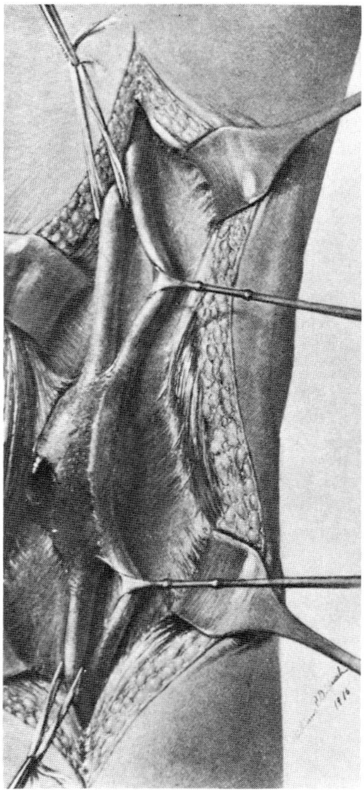

Figure 6. This illustration is taken from the report of Bernheim and shows a popliteal aneurysm densely adherent to the popliteal vein. A small area of the sac wall is shown which was quite thin and the author thought represented an area of threatened rupture. The following three illustrations (Figs. 7, 8, and 9) are also taken from the original paper by Bernheim. (Bull. of The Johns Hopkins Hospital, 27: 93, 1916.)

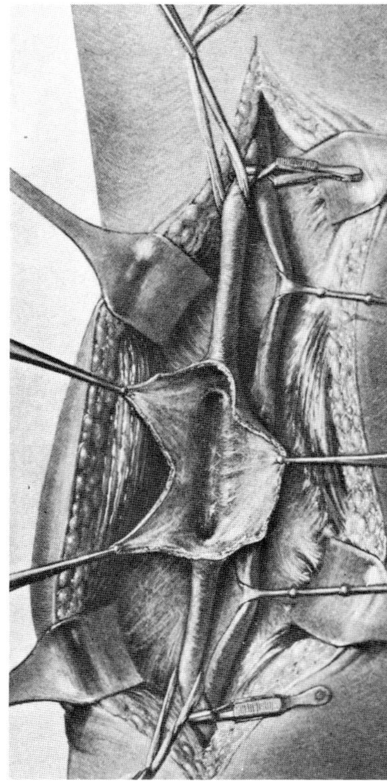

Figure 7. The aneurysmal sac was opened, demonstrating the entrance and exit of the popliteal artery above and below. (Bull. of The Johns Hopkins Hospital, 27: 93, 1916.)

generally accompanied by classical symptoms of angina pectoris, of marked electrocardiographic changes during exercise, and often with the presence of calcium observed radiologically in the region of this vessel. Most patients experience complete relief of pain and improved survival following myocardial revascularization. In patients in whom symptoms of

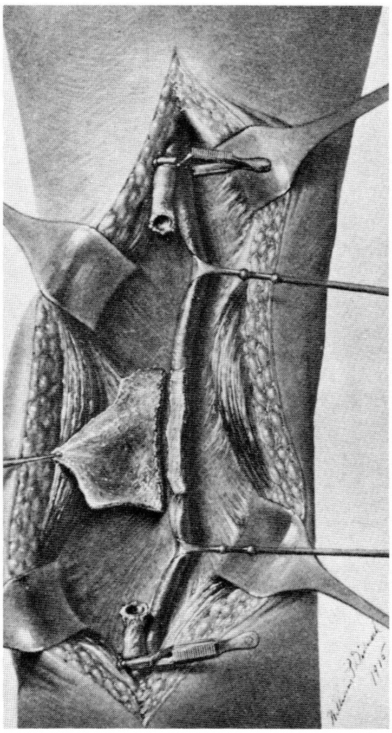

Figure 8. Following dissection of the popliteal aneurysm, very little of the wall ultimately remained, thus leaving the two ends of the popliteal artery widely apart. (Bull. of The Johns Hopkins Hospital, 27: 93, 1916.)

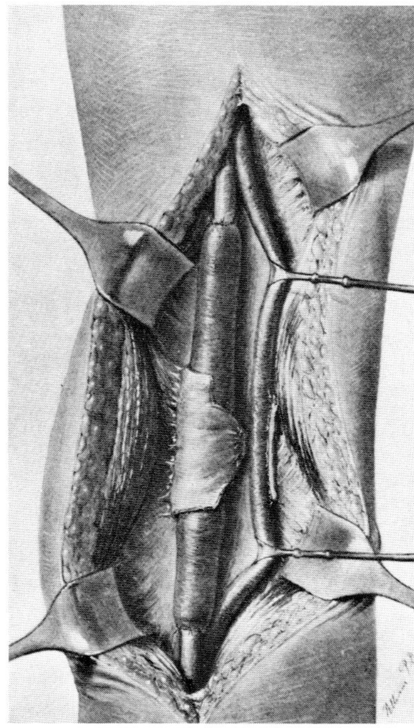

Figure 9. A segment of saphenous vein autograft was removed and sutured end-to-end as shown here. A portion of the aneurysmal wall was wrapped around it in an attempt to provide reinforcement of the thin walled vein graft. (Bull. of The Johns Hopkins Hospital, 27: 93, 1916.)

pre-infarction angina are present, the clinical situation should usually be considered a surgical emergency. Revascularization procedures for this serious lesion have been associated with a continuously diminishing mortality and should be performed for proper management of this condition.

## REFERENCES

1. Cohen, M. V., Cohn, P. F., Herman, M. V., and Gorlin, R. 1972. Diagnosis and prognosis of main left coronary obstruction. Circulation, Suppl. 1, 45 and 46: 57.
2. Lavine, P., Kimbiris, D., Segal, B. L., and Linhart, J. W. 1972. Left

main coronary artery disease. Clinical, arteriographic and hemodynamic appraisal. Am. J. Cardiol. 30: 791.
3. Bruschke, A. V. G., Proudfit, W. L., and Sones, F. M., Jr. 1973. Progress study of 590 consecutive nonsurgical cases of coronary disease followed 5–9 years. I. Arteriographic correlations. Circulation 47: 1147.
4. James, T. N. 1961. Anatomy of the Coronary Arteries. Paul B. Hoeber, Inc., New York.
5. Zeft, H. J., Manley, J. C., Huston, J. H., Tector, A. J., Auer, J. E., and Johnson, W. D. 1974. Left main coronary artery stenosis. Results of coronary bypass surgery. Circulation 49: 68.
6. Khaja, F-U., Sharma, S. D., Easley, R. M., Jr., Heinle, R. A., and Goldstein, S. 1974. Left main coronary artery lesions. Risks of catheterization; exercise testing and surgery. Circulation, Suppl. 2, 49 and 50: 136.
7. Kisslo, J. (personal communication).
8. Bartel, A. G., Behar, V. S., Peter, R. H., Orgain, E. S., and Kong, Y. 1974. Graded exercise stress tests in angiographically documented coronary artery disease. Circulation 49: 348.
9. Pichard, A. D., Sheldon, W. C., Shinji, K., Effler, D. B., and Sones, F. M., Jr. 1973. Severe arteriosclerotic obstruction of the left main coronary artery: Follow-up results in 176 patients. Circulation, Suppl. 4, 7, and 8: 53.
10. Brymer, J. F., Buter, T. H., Walton, J. A., Jr., and Willis, P. W., III. 1974. A natural history study of the prognostic role of coronary arteriography. Am. Heart J. 88: 139.
11. Herrick, J. B. 1912. Clinical features of sudden obstruction of the coronary arteries. JAMA 59: 2015.
12. Fraentzel: Krankheiten des Herzens, Berlin, 1892, iii, 51. Cited in Herrick, J. B. 1912. Clinical features of sudden obstruction of the coronary arteries. JAMA 59: 2015.
13. Heberden, W. 1818. Commentaries on the History and Cure of Diseases, p. 292. Wells and Lilly, Boston.
14. Osler, W. 1897. Lectures on Angina Pectoris and Allied States. D. Appleton & Co., New York.
15. Sabiston, D. C., Jr. 1974. The coronary circulation. The William F. Rienhoff, Jr. Lecture. Johns Hopkins Med. J. 134: 314.
16. Goyanes, D. J. 1906. Substitution plastica de las arterias por las venas, o arterioplastia venosa, aplicada, como nuevo metodo, al tratamiento de los aneurismas. El Siglo Medico, Sept. 1, pp. 346–348; Sept. 8, pp. 561–564.
17. Lexer, E. 1907. Die ideale Operation des arteriellen und des Arteriellvenosen Aneurysma. Archiv. f. klin. Chir. 83: 459.
18. Bernheim, B. M. 1916. The ideal operation for aneurisms of the extremity. Report of a case. Bull. Johns Hopkins Hosp. 27: 93.
19. Murray, G., Porcheron, R., Hilario, J., and Roschlau, W. 1954. Anastomosis of a systemic artery to the coronary. Canad. Med. Assoc. J. 71: 594.
20. Garrett, H. E., Dennis, E. W., and DeBakey, M. E. 1973. Aortocoronary bypass with saphenous vein graft. Seven-year follow-up. JAMA 223: 792.

21. Favaloro, R. G. 1968. Saphenous vein autograft replacement of severe segmental coronary artery occlusion. Operative technique. Ann. Thorac. Surg. 5: 334.
22. Johnson, W. D., Flemma, R. J., Lepley, D., Jr., and Ellison, E. H. 1969. Extended treatment of severe coronary artery disease. A total surgical approach. Ann. Surg. 170: 460.

# 2
# Pre-Infarction Angina in Left Main Coronary Artery Disease

P. J. Scanlon, M.D., J. V. Talano, M.D.,
R. Nemickas, M.D., R. Pifarre, M.D.,
J. M. Moran, M.D., and R. M. Gunnar, M.D.

Obstruction of the left main coronary artery (LCA) is now known to be a critical anatomical defect. Several reports, including our own, have pointed out a high incidence of unstable or pre-infarction angina (PIA) in patients with LCA disease (1–4). Because we suspected that patients with LCA disease who have unstable angina have a worse prognosis than those with more stable clinical states, we have compared our clinical, hemodynamic, angiographic and therapeutic experiences in these two groups of patients. The findings of these comparisons form the basis of this report.

## DEFINITIONS

Left main coronary disease was defined as 50% or greater obstruction of this vessel as seen angiographically.

Significant obstruction of other major coronary vessels was defined as at least 70% obstruction of those vessels as seen angiographically.

Left ventricular dysfunction was defined as dyskinesia, akinesia and/or severe hypokinesia of at least 50% of the ventricular outline, or a ventricular aneurysm as seen in the right anterior oblique projection during left ventricular angiography.

Pre-infarction angina was defined as a recent progressive increase in the severity, duration, and/or frequency of angina pectoris without electrocardiographic or enzymatic changes of myocardial infarction.

## CLINICAL MATERIAL

From January 1, 1970 to February 1, 1974, approximately 1500 patients with coronary artery disease were studied by coronary arteriography at Loyola University Medical Center. Of these, 107 patients were found to have LCA disease. Pre-infarction angina was the presenting problem in 46 patients (43%), whereas 55 patients had stable angina. Four patients presented with dyspnea on exertion without angina, and one patient was studied because of severe recurrent ventricular arrhythmias. The latter 61 patients make up the "stable" group for purposes of this report. The mean follow-up period was 18 months.

The clinical characteristics of the two groups of patients are presented in Table I. There was no significant difference regarding sex distribution or age. The patients with PIA had a duration of angina of 37.3 ± 7.5 months (mean ± SE), much shorter than the 57.0 ± 6.8 months for the stable group. In 89% of the PIA group there was a recent history of rest pain whereas only 41% of the stable group had rest pain ($p < 0.001$). Both groups had a high incidence of old myocardial infarction (56% with PIA versus 51% in stable patients). A history of congestive heart failure was especially frequent in both groups, occurring in 24% of PIA patients, and in 23% of stable patients. There was no significant difference between the two groups in relation to the incidence of the coronary risk factors, i.e., hypertension, diabetes, or heavy smoking (one pack or more). Physical findings in the two groups of patients were also similar.

The period of unstable angina in the pre-infarction group ranged from 1 to 90 days, with a mean of 24.3 days.

Table I. Clinical Characteristics of 107 Patients with LMC Disease

| | PIA Group | Stable Group |
|---|---|---|
| Patients | 46 | 61 |
| Males | 38 | 52 |
| Females | 8 | 9 |
| Age | 55.2 ± 1.2 | 54.7 ± 0.9 |
| Months of angina | 37.3 ± 7.5 | 57.0 ± 6.8 |
| Rest pain | 89% | 41% |
| Congestive failure | 24% | 23% |
| Old infarction | 56% | 51% |
| Hypertension | 30% | 21% |
| Diabetes | 11% | 5% |
| Smokers | 50% | 56% |

## HEMODYNAMIC DATA

Right heart catheterization was performed in 103 patients, and left heart catheterization was performed in all 107 patients. We have reported previously that several hemodynamic abnormalities suggest a poor long-term prognosis in patients with pre-infarction angina (5). These abnormalities are: left ventricular end diastolic pressure (LVEDP) >12 mm. Hg, cardiac index <2.7 L/min./m.$^2$, stroke index <35 cc./beat/m.$^2$, estimated cardiac work (mean aortic pressure × cardiac index) <240 units, and left ventricular ejection fraction <50%. In this study the two clinical groups were compared in relation to the degree and frequency of these hemodynamic abnormalities. A pulmonary artery systolic pressure >30 mm. Hg was an additional abnormality studied.

Table II reveals that hemodynamic abnormalities were common in both PIA patients and stable patients. There were no significant differences between the two groups in relation to the mean value of any hemodynamic variable or in relation to the frequency of any hemodynamic abnormality among patients within the two groups. For example, mean LVEDP was 16.0 mm. Hg for PIA patients and 16.2 mm. Hg for stable patients, and 58% of PIA patients and 57% of stable patients had an abnormal LVEDP.

Table II. Hemodynamic Characteristics of 107 Patients with LMC Disease

| | PIA Group (46) | Stable Group (61) |
|---|---|---|
| LVEDP | 16.0 ± 1.5 | 16.2 ± 1.1 |
| % > 12 mm. Hg | 58% | 57% |
| Cardiac index | 2.57 ± 0.1 | 2.59 ± 0.1 |
| % < 2.7 L/min./m.$^2$ | 43% | 53% |
| Stroke index | 32.9 ± 1.5 | 33.6 ± 1.4 |
| % < 35 cc./beat/m.$^2$ | 57% | 61% |
| Cardiac work | 258 ± 12.9 | 248 ± 10.5 |
| % < 240 units | 37% | 44% |
| Ejection fraction | 44.4 ± 3.3 | 41.3 ± 3.4 |
| % < 50% | 48% | 58% |
| Pulmonary systolic | 30.6 ± 2.1 | 32.3 ± 2.0 |
| % > 30 mm. Hg | 35% | 33% |

## ANGIOGRAPHIC DATA

Coronary arteriography was performed by the Sones technique in 97 patients, Judkins technique in 9 patients, and both techniques in 1 patient. Multiple vessel disease was found in the vast majority of both clinical groups of LCA disease patients (Table III). Seventy-six percent of PIA patients and 77% of stable patients had significant obstruction of at least three major coronary arteries, including the LCA. The right coronary artery was significantly obstructed in 74% of the PIA group and in 80% of the stable group, and the left anterior descending was obstructed in 70% of the former and 72% of the latter. The LCA was completely obstructed in one patient with PIA and in two stable patients. Three patients in each clinical group had obstruction only in the LCA. Intercoronary collaterals were visualized in 71% of the stable patients and in 63% of PIA patients. This difference was not significant.

Major ventricular contraction abnormalities were present in the majority of patients in both groups (70% of PIA group and 67% of the stable group). Ventricular aneurysms were more common in the stable group (20% versus 12.5%), although not significantly so. One patient in the stable group had a post-myocardial infarction ventricular septal defect.

Complications within 24 hr. of catheterization were uncommon. Of the PIA group, one patient had ventricular tachycardia of brief duration during study. Another suffered an acute myocardial infarction 6 hr. after catheterization and died 24 hr. later. Another patient sustained an infarction 4 hr. after study, and was successfully operated on as an emergency. Of the stable group, one patient whose presenting complaint was congestive heart failure died immediately after study. Three others had ventricu-

Table III. Angiographic Findings in 107 Patients with LMC Disease

| | PIA Group (46) (%) | Stable Group (61) (%) |
|---|---|---|
| Number of obstructed vessels | | |
| 1 | 7 | 5 |
| 2 | 17 | 18 |
| 3 | 17 | 20 |
| >3 | 59 | 57 |
| Collaterals | 62 | 71 |
| Major ventricular abnormalities | 70 | 67 |
| Ventricular aneurysms | 12.5 | 20 |

lar fibrillation during the procedure; all were successfully resuscitated. One patient suffered a cerebral vascular accident. Another patient died suddenly 18 hr. after uneventful catheterization, presumably because of a ventricular arrhythmia. Thus, the risk of catheterization was no different for PIA patients than for stable patients with LCA disease.

## TREATMENT

Management of both clinical groups of patients was of three types.

Thirty-four (74%) of the 46 patients in the PIA group and 40 (66%) of the 61 stable patients underwent surgery. The only major clinical differences between the two surgical groups were the shorter duration of angina (35.3 ± 8.5 months versus 53.6 ± 7.6 months), and the higher frequency of rest pain (88% versus 50%, $p < 0.001$) in the PIA group. Hemodynamically and angiographically there were no significant differences.

Four PIA patients (8.7%) and 14 stable patients (23%) were considered operable angiographically, but for various reasons did not undergo surgery. These two groups were clinically comparable except for more frequent rest pain (100% versus 13%, $p < 0.001$) and a more frequent history of previous myocardial infarction (75% versus 33%, NS), in patients with PIA. Both groups had more frequent and more severe hemodynamic abnormalities than did their operated counterparts, but there were no major hemodynamic or angiographic differences between the two non-operated groups.

Eight of the PIA group (17%) and six of the stable patients (9.8%) were considered inoperable angiographically and so were treated medically. The PIA group was older (60.5 ± 2.2 years versus 52.7 ± 3.1 years) than the stable group, but their mean duration of angina was shorter (37.1 ± 2.09 months versus 72.0 ∓ 24.4 months). Eighty-eight percent of the PIA group had rest pain, versus 50% of the stable patients. The stable group had greater hemodynamic impairment than the PIA group. Fifty percent of the stable inoperable patients had a ventricular aneurysm, whereas only 12.5% of the PIA patients had an aneurysm (NS), perhaps partially explaining the higher frequency of hemodynamic abnormalities in the former group.

The inoperable patients of both groups were sicker than their operated counterparts. Clinically the inoperable groups had much higher incidences of congestive heart failure (43% versus 11%, $p < 0.001$), and of diabetes mellitis (29% versus 4%, $p < 0.001$). These differences were reflected in the more frequent hemodynamic abnormalities, in the more diffuse nature of the coronary disease, and in the higher frequency of ventricular contraction abnormalities in inoperable patients. Because of these differences it is impossible to compare accurately the outcome of treatment among the three management groups.

## RESULTS OF TREATMENT

In hospital surgical mortality was 15% (5 of 34) for the PIA group and 7.5% (3 of 40) for the stable group (Table IV). There were two late deaths in the former group for a total mortality of 21%, and one late death in the latter group for an overall mortality of 10%. These death rates were not significantly different statistically. Four of the PIA group were operated on during the acute phase of a myocardial infarction, with two deaths, whereas only two of the stable group had surgery during acute infarction, with one death.

Of the 27 PIA patients who survived surgery, 20 are now angina-free (74%). Five others have mild angina, one moderate angina, and another severe angina. Ninety-three percent of the survivors, representing 73% of all PIA patients who went to surgery, are significantly improved. Of the 36 stable patients surviving surgery, 30 are angina free (83%). Four others have mild pain, one moderate angina, and one severe angina. Ninety-four percent of the survivors, representing 85% of all stable patients undergoing surgery are significantly improved. These differences are not statistically significant.

Of the four operable PIA patients treated medically, two died within 2 weeks, both of acute myocardial infarction. Of the 14 operable stable patients treated medically, six died (43%), one suddenly 18 hr. after study, four within 3 months, and one 2 years later. Of the two PIA survivors, one

Table IV. Follow-up in 74 LCA Patients Treated Surgically

| | PIA Group (34 Patients) | Stabel Group (40 Patients) |
|---|---|---|
| Deaths | | |
| Early | 5 (15%) | 3 (7.5%) |
| Total | 7 (21%) | 4 (10%) |
| Survivors - total | 27 (79%) | 36 (90%) |
| Mild angina | 5 | 4 |
| Moderate angina | 1 | 1 |
| Severe angina | 1 | 1 |
| Asymptomatic | 20 (59%) | 30 (75%) |

has moderate angina; of the eight stable survivors, one is symptom free, three have mild angina, one has severe angina, and three have chronic congestive heart failure. Thus, of the operable group treated medically, one of four PIA patients, and only four of 14 stable patients are improved (Table V).

Of the eight inoperable PIA patients, four died (50%), three within 1 week, following acute myocardial infarction, and one suddenly 3 months later. Of the six inoperable stable patients, three died during follow-up, all within 2 months, and all of congestive heart failure. All four PIA survivors continue to have angina, although two are improved. Two of the stable survivors have mild angina, and one continues to have severe pain. Of the entire inoperable group, only two of eight PIA patients are improved, and only two of six patients in the stable group are improved.

Of 46 LCA patients with PIA, nine (20%) actually suffered a near-term acute myocardial infarction. Five of these patients died with their infarction, and four others had emergency surgery, with two deaths. Of the 61 stable patients, only three (5%) suffered an early myocardial infarction; one died the same day and two went to emergency surgery, with one death. This difference in the near-term infarction rate is statistically significant ($p < 0.05$).

Previously we reported that a history of congestive heart failure, or the finding of any of five hemodynamic abnormalities as discussed above, were associated with a significantly increased risk of death in patients with PIA. Similar risks were noted in the two clinical groups in this study, but there was no difference in the risks between the two groups. For example, 73% of 11 PIA patients with congestive heart failure died and 64% of 14 stable patients with congestive failure died, whereas the mortality rates for the two groups in the absence of congestive heart failure were only 14% ($p <$

Table V. Follow-up in 32 LMC Patients Treated Medically

| | Operable | | Inoperable | |
|---|---|---|---|---|
| | PIA (4 Patients) | Stable (14 Patients) | PIA (8 Patients) | Stable (6 Patients) |
| Deaths | 2 (50%) | 6 (43%) | 4 (50%) | 3 (50%) |
| Survivors | 2 (50%) | 8 (57%) | 4 (50%) | 3 (50%) |
| Mild angina | 0 | 3 | 1 | 2 |
| Moderate angina | 1 | 0 | 1 | 0 |
| Severe angina | 0 | 1 | 2 | 1 |
| Congestive failure | 0 | 3 | 0 | 0 |
| Asymptomatic | 1 | 1 | 0 | 0 |

0.001) and 11% ($p < 0.001$) respectively. We could discover no parameter which presented significant risk for the PIA group but not for the stable group, or vice versa.

## DISCUSSION

Our incidence of pre-infarction angina in patients with LCA disease was similar to the 47% incidence of accelerating angina reported by Lavine et al. (1). This is the first attempt to compare patients with LCA disease who present with PIA with those without this anginal pattern.

Except for the anginal pattern there was very little clinical difference between the two groups. The fact that the mean duration of angina was 20 months shorter in the PIA group indicates a generally more rapid deterioration for the group, but does not explain why PIA occurs. The higher incidence of rest pain in PIA patients would be expected, as it is part of the unstable angina syndrome and many authors include rest pain as a prerequisite for the diagnosis of PIA.

Cardiac catheterization and coronary and left ventricular angiography can be carried out at an acceptable risk, although earlier reports suggested that the risk might be prohibitive. There was no greater risk for patients with PIA than for stable patients with LCA disease. The hemodynamic and angiographic findings at catheterization did not significantly differ between the two groups. The majority of both groups had severe multiple vessel coronary disease and significant impairment of left ventricular function.

The results of treatment of LCA disease suggest that surgery carries a higher risk for patients who present with PIA than for more stable patients, although there were not enough patients in our study for this difference to be statistically significant. Survivors of surgery did equally well regardless of their preoperative anginal state.

Medically treated patients did much worse than surgically treated patients with LCA disease, although the medical group was clinically sicker and had more frequent hemodynamic and angiographic abnormalities than the surgical group. There was no difference between the outcome in medically treated patients with PIA and those with stable symptoms.

The term "pre-infarction angina" appears to be somewhat justified by the finding that a significantly greater number of PIA group suffered near-term infarction (20%) than did the stable group (5%) ($p < 0.05$). The number of infarctions would probably have been greater if early surgery had not been performed in the majority of patients in both groups.

## REFERENCES

1. Lavine, P., Kimbiris, D., Segal, B. L., and Linhart, J. W. 1972. Left main coronary artery disease. Am. J. Cardiol. 30: 791.
2. Cohen, M. V., Cohn, P. F., Herman, M. V., and Gorlin, R. 1972. Diagnosis and prognosis of main left coronary artery obstruction. Circulation 45 (Suppl I): 57.
3. Scanlon, P. J., Talano, J. V., Moran, J. F., and Gunnar, R. M. 1974. Main left coronary artery disease. Am. J. Cardiol. 33: 169.
4. Talano, J. V., Scanlon, P. J., Khan, M., Meadows, W. R., Loeb, H. S., Pifarre, R., and Gunnar, R. M. Influence of surgery on survival in 145 patients with left main coronary artery disease. Circulation (In press).
5. Scanlon, P. J., Nemickas, R., Moran, J. F., Talano, J. V., Amirparviz, F., and Pifarre, R. 1973. Accelerated angina pectoris: clinical, hemodynamic, arteriographic and therapeutic experience in 85 patients. Circulation 47: 19.

# 3
# Angiographic Diagnosis of Left Main Coronary Artery Disease

R. E. Falicov, M.D.

Ever since the introduction by Sones as a clinically feasible, generally safe diagnostic procedure, selective coronary arteriography has continued to gain increased acceptance throughout the world as the most accurate procedure available for the anatomical evaluation of obstructive coronary arterial disease. It is estimated that 400,000 coronary arteriographic procedures are performed in the world yearly (1). Through the widespread use of coronary arteriography, rapid advances have been made in the last decade in the understanding of the natural history of coronary arterial disease, and its modification by different therapeutic modalities, mainly surgical interventions.

## ANGIOGRAPHIC DIAGNOSIS OF LEFT MAIN CORONARY ARTERY DISEASE

The incidence of significant left main coronary artery stenosis (LMCAS) (more than 50% luminal obstruction) among patients having angiographic evidence of coronary artery disease is estimated between 5 and 10% (2–3). Analysis of several series recently reported (3–6) reveals several clinical and laboratory clues that may lead to the suspicion that significant LMCAS will be found on arteriographic examination, the most common being a presentation of unstable or crescendo angina pectoris, the presence of dyspnea in association with angina, and severe S-T segment depression (more than 2 mm.) during treadmill exercise testing. Recently, significant arterial hypotension during treadmill exercise testing (7) has also been found strongly correlated with the presence of LMCAS or other proximal, critical coronary artery narrowings. On the other hand there have been no unequivocal correlates of LMCAS (8), and hence the lesions still may be found in the absence of any of these clinical or electrocardiographic clues (Table I).

Patients with severe LMCAS appeared to be at a significantly increased risk. Mortality in connection with diagnostic coronary arteriography in patients with LMCAS has been reported higher than the average mortality risk of the procedure, estimated from large series to be approximately 0.5% (9). The highest figure (5 deaths in a series of 32 patients, or 15%) was reported in 1972 by Cohen and co-workers (3). Three of these five deaths occurred by cardiac arrest within 10 sec. of introducing a preformed catheter (Judkins) into the left coronary ostium, while the other two fatalities resulted from myocardial infarction and occurred 1 and 15 days after the procedure in patients studied with the Sones technique. Other more recent series (4–6, 8, 10) have had lower mortality figures in connection with diagnostic catheterization and angiography (Table II). In any case, it seems clear that patients having severe LMCAS are particularly labile, tolerate hemodynamic disturbances poorly, and should be dealt with utmost care.

In our laboratory, we follow an established technique with the aim of obtaining as complete a diagnostic study as possible while at the same time trying to prevent possible complications. After the preformed left coronary Judkins catheter has been introduced percutaneously via the femoral artery into the aortic arch, it is flushed vigorously, and 50 mg. of sodium heparin administered through the catheter. The catheter is then filled with angiographic contrast material, and the patient is positioned in a 30° left anterior oblique position. The left coronary artery ostium is located approximately 30° posteriorly in relation to the frontal plane (Fig. 1A). Hence a 30° left anterior oblique projection will display the coronary

| Table I. Clues to the Presence of Left Main Coronary Artery Stenosis |
|---|
| Unstable or crescendo angina |
| Dyspnea with angina |
| Multistage treadmill exercise test |
| > 2 mm. S-T depression |
| Hypotension during M.S.E.T. |
| None of the above |

Table II. Left Main Coronary Artery Stenosis Mortality

| Group (No. of Pts.) | Arteriography (%) | Medical ℞ (Follow-up) | Surgical ℞ Early | Surgical ℞ Late |
|---|---|---|---|---|
| Brushke et al. (37) | 0 | 57% (5 yr.) | | |
| Cohen et al. (32) | 15 | 50% (25 mo.) | 29% | |
| Lavine et al. (30) | 10 | 33% (1 mo.) | 11% | |
| Talano et al. (145) | 3 | 54% (1 yr.) | 27% (1 yr.) | |
| Pichard et al. (176) | 0.7 | 26% (3 yr.) | 8% | 39% (1 yr.) |
| Kisslo et al. (52) | 2 | 25% (1 yr.) | 39% | 39% (1 yr.) |
| Khaja et al. (28) | 0 | | 28% | 0 (18 mo.) |

ostium and proximal left main coronary artery in full profile and allow the diagnosis of proximal LMCAS (Fig. 1B). Figure 1C illustrates the fact that a steep right anterior oblique position will hide the proximal left main coronary artery from view and thus if this projection is employed initially significant LMCAS can be overlooked.

As the catheter approaches the left coronary sinus of Valsalva in the 30° left anterior oblique position, contrast material is injected manually to locate the left coronary ostium. A vigorous injection of contrast material while the catheter tip is confronting the left coronary ostium will visualize the proximal portions of the left coronary tree and thus a severe ostial or proximal left main coronary lesion can usually be diagnosed from this nonselective injection. If the proximal main artery is clear, the ostium is next engaged in the usual manner and the study proceeds to completion by obtaining six views of the left coronary tree in different degrees of obliquity. If, on the other hand, a proximal lesion is visualized from the nonselective injection, the subsequent course of the study is modified as follows.

While pressure is being monitored continuously, the catheter is advanced very gently a few millimeters into the ostium. If the pressure waveform dampens, the catheter is immediately withdrawn and only nonselective sinus injections performed. If the pressure waveform remains undamped, a short injection of contrast medium is filmed coming down on the proximal left coronary tree in the 30° left anterior oblique position. If the proximal stenosis is confirmed from this injection, the next injection is then filmed in the 20° right anterior oblique projection, which allows good visualization of the middle and distal portions of the main left coronary artery as well as the origin of the left anterior descending coronary artery. If these two injections are well tolerated by the patient, we complete the

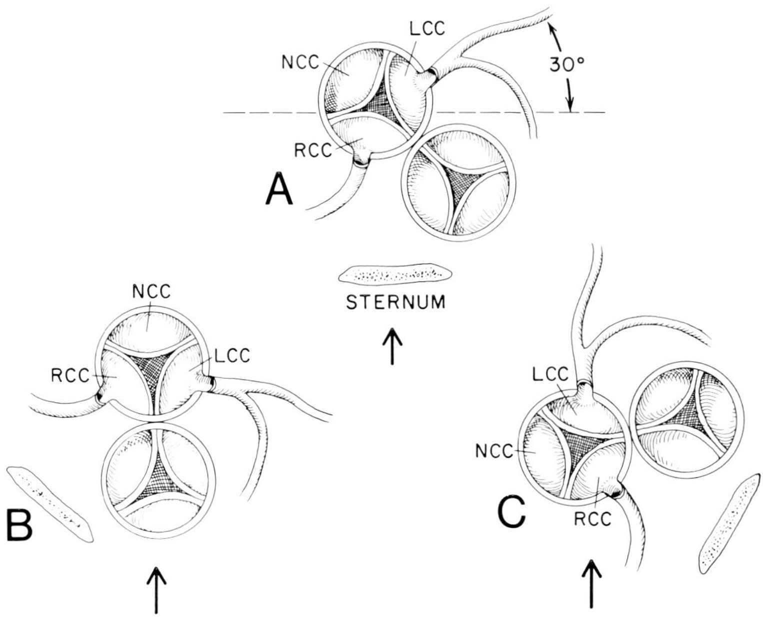


Figure 1. A. Schematic representation of the aortic root with the origin of the coronary arteries as seen from above. The main left coronary artery is oriented 30° posteriorly from the frontal plane. B. When the patient is in a 30° left anterior oblique position the main left coronary artery and the origin of the circumflex coronary artery are in full profile. This is the preferred view for the first injection into the LMCA. C. 60° right anterior oblique position. The ostium and proximal LMCA are hidden from view. The proximal left anterior descending artery is now in full profile.

visualization of the left coronary tree with injections in a 60° right and 60° left anterior oblique projections.

The following precautions are observed in every coronary arteriographic procedure performed in our laboratory, and become particularly important when studying a patient with severe, proximal disease or who is clinically unstable: 1) Anticoagulation with 50 mg. of sodium heparin at the start of the study, followed by neutralization by protamine sulphate before the last catheter is removed. 2) Administration of atropine sulphate (0.5 to 2 mg.) as needed to avoid bradycardia and vasovagal reactions. 3) Continuous monitoring of blood pressure and two leads of the electrocardiogram. 4) If a patient develops anginal pain at any moment during the study, the procedure is halted and oxygen by mask and sublingual nitroglycerine 0.4 mg. given, and repeated as needed until the pain ceases. 5) Coronary injections are performed only while the patient is totally pain-free and the electrocardiogram has returned to baseline levels if it has been altered by a previous injection.

Occasionally, coronary arterial narrowing may be caused by arterial spasm. There is substantial evidence now available that coronary spasm may play an essential role in the pathogenesis of the so-called variant, or Prinzmetal angina (11, 12). Proximal spasm may be spontaneous, or induced by contact with the catheter tip. Hence, if proximal narrowing is observed during filming, particularly if smooth and tapered, the injection should be repeated in the same projection after the administration of sublingual nitroglycerine. An example of spasm of the left main coronary artery is illustrated in Figure 2. The detection of a spastic component to coronary arterial disease has important therapeutic implications, since the results of bypass graft surgery in patients with an important spastic component to their coronary disease have generally been disappointing (11, 12).

Significant LMCAS is as a rule associated with severe, widespread coronary occlusive lesions and indicates advanced atherosclerosis (13). This is exemplified in the following case.

## Case 1

A 59-year-old man developed chest pain on exertion in 1966, followed shortly by an acute myocardial infarction from which he recovered uneventfully. His angina returned and continued stable for the next 8 years until April of 1974 when he noticed a definite increase in the frequency of pains which did not respond to therapy with propranolol and long-acting nitrites. Recently, he had developed dyspnea associated with angina. In 1973 he had a sudden loss of vision in the right eye, and underwent carotid endarterectomy for severe stenosis of the right carotid artery. Physical examination revealed a right carotid bruit, bilateral nasocanthal xanthelasma, and an enlarged, dyskinetic left ventricular impulse with a palpable and audible atrial sound. Serum cholesterol was 450 mg.%, serum triglycerides were 260 mg.%. Heavy calcification was noted in his proximal left coronary artery during fluoroscopy. Coronary arteriography (Fig. 3) revealed a severe, diffuse narrowing of his left main coronary artery; in addition he had multiple obstructive lesions of the left anterior descending coronary artery. Both branches of the circumflex coronary artery were occluded and filled by collaterals from both the left anterior descending and the right coronary arteries. The right coronary artery had several areas of narrowing. A left ventriculogram revealed a diffusely hypokinetic ventricle with an ejection fraction of 0.42. The patient underwent double

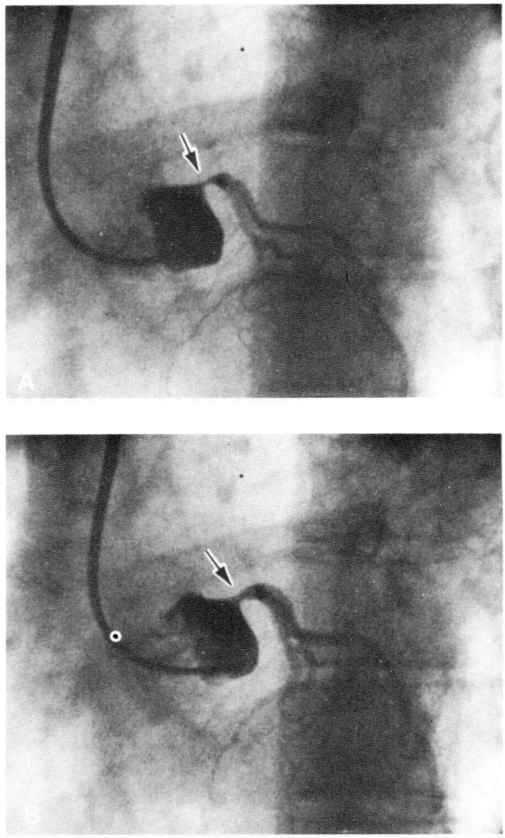


Figure 2. A. Shallow left anterior oblique projection of a coronary sinus injection outlining severe stenosis of the proximal LMCA. The smooth contour of the stenotic segment suggests arterial spasm. B. Repeated sinus injection in the same projection after sublingual nitroglycerine. The stenosis has become much less severe. (Courtesy of Drs. H. Lardani and F. Mason Sones, Jr.).

bypass graft to the mid-portion of the left anterior descending and the atrioventricular branch of the circumflex coronary arteries. Postoperatively he did very well, with marked decrease in anginal attacks but died suddenly while gardening 6 months after surgery.

Occasionally a critical lesion of the left main coronary artery can be isolated as shown in the following case.

## Case 2

A 39-year-old man noticed retrosternal discomfort 2 years previously while exerting. He responded well to nitroglycerine and beta adrenergic

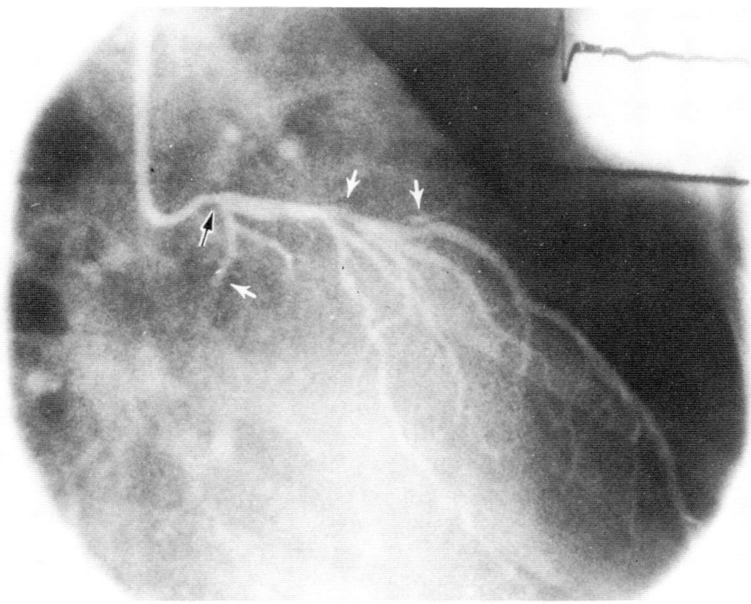

Figure 3. Shallow right anterior oblique projection of a left coronary artery injection in Case 1. There is severe stenosis of the LMCA (black arrow). In addition, the left anterior descending artery has several areas of stenosis and the circumflex artery is occluded (white arrows).

blockade, but continued to have two to three episodes of exertional angina per month. There was no resting or nocturnal angina. Physical examination was essentially negative with exception of a slight arcus senilis. The resting electrocardiogram was within normal limits, but a treadmill multistage exercise test revealed marked S-T depression (4 mm.) in the precordial leads during exercise and early recovery phase. Coronary arteriography revealed severe stenosis of the middle and distal portions of the main left coronary artery involving the origin of both the left anterior descending and circumflex coronary arteries (Fig. 4). The rest of the left coronary tree showed no abnormalities. The circumflex was dominant and supplied the inferior wall of the left ventricle. The right coronary artery was small and showed no abnormalities. The left ventricle contracted symmetrically and vigorously. The patient underwent saphenous vein bypass graft to both the mid-left anterior descending and the circumflex coronary arteries. Recovery was uneventful; the patient has been symptom-free, and back to work 2 years postoperatively.

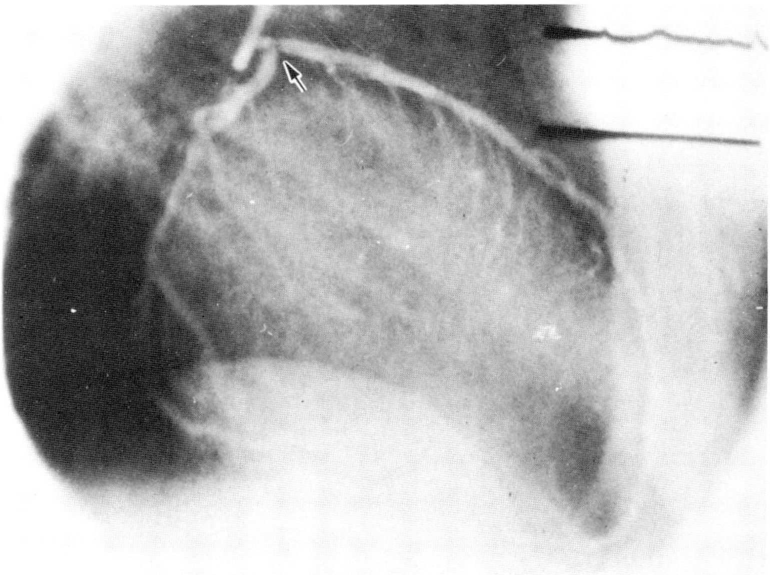

Figure 4. Shallow right anterior oblique projection of a left coronary artery injection in Case 2. There is high grade stenosis of the distal LMCA involving the origins of both the anterior descending and circumflex branches. The circumflex is dominant and supplies the inferior wall of the ventricles. Both branches of the LMCA are smooth and free of obstructions.

Table II summarizes mortality figures within a given follow-up time of some of the recently reported series of patients with LMCAS. As it can be appreciated from these figures, the prognosis in this group of patients appears relatively poor, regardless of whether or not bypass surgery is performed. Mention is made in some of the reports, however, that in patients surviving the operation symptoms are considerably lessened and the quality of life improved. Our recent experience with patients having LMCAS at the University of Chicago agrees with this general overview. Eight patients with LMCAS were studied between October 1973 and November 1974, with an average follow-up of 5 months. All underwent arteriography without complications, and all survived surgery, one being complicated by sternal dehiscence. At the time of this writing, one patient has died 6 months postoperatively (Case 1 reported above), and of seven survivors, four have completed convalescence and returned to their occupation markedly improved, while the other three are still convalescing; none have significant angina pectoris.

## SUMMARY AND CONCLUSIONS

Stenosis of the left main coronary artery is as a rule a manifestation of, and is associated with, severe, generalized atherosclerotic involvement of the coronary arterial tree. Clinical clues to the presence of LMCAS include unstable or crescendo angina pectoris, dyspnea associated with angina, and severe abnormalities in the exercise electrocardiogram, but it can be present without any of these indicators. Mortality associated with the arteriographic diagnosis of LMCAS, which was high a few years ago, has decreased considerably, most likely because of the increased recognition of the lability of these patients which has resulted in a more cautious attitude during arteriography. The femoral approach can be safely used if precautions are properly taken. The long-term prognosis of patients with left main coronary artery stenosis is relatively poor, regardless of whether or not bypass surgery is performed, but successful surgery appears to bring relief of symptoms and improve the quality of life in a substantial number of these patients.

## REFERENCES

1. Wholey, M. H. 1974. Clinical dosimetry during the angiographic examination: Comments on coronary arteriography. Circulation 50: 627–631.
2. Proudfit, W. L., Shirey, E. K., and Sones, F. M. Jr. 1967. Distribution of arterial lesions demonstrated by selective cinecoronary arteriography. Circulation 36: 54.
3. Cohen, M. V., Cohn, P. F., Herman, M. V., and Gorlin, R. 1972. Diagnosis and prognosis of main left coronary artery obstruction. Circulation 35–36:(Suppl. I)I, 57–65.
4. Khaja, F. U., Sherman, S. D., Easley, R. M. Jr., Heinle, R. A., and Goldstein, S. 1974. Left main coronary artery lesions: Risks of catheterization, exercise testing and surgery. Circulation 49–50 (Suppl. II): II, 136–140.
5. Lavine, P., Kimbiris, D., Segal, B. L., and Linhart, J. W. Left main coronary artery disease: Clinical, arteriographic and hemodynamic appraisal. Am. J. Cardiol. 30: 791–796.
6. Battock, D. J., Steele, P. P., and Davies, H. 1974. Left main coronary artery disease: Is surgery always indicated? Am. J. Cardiol. 33: 125. (Abstr).
7. Thomson, P. D. and Kelemen, M. H. 1974. A reliable and easily elicited sign of critical coronary artery narrowing. Circulation 49–50 (Suppl): III-9. (Abstr.).
8. Kisslo, J., Peter, R., Behar, V., Bartel, A., and Kong, Y. 1973. Left main coronary artery stenosis. Circulation 47–48 (Suppl. IV): IV-57. (Abstr.).

9. Adams, D. F., Fraser, D. B., and Abrams, H. L. The complications of coronary arteriography. Circulation 48: 609.
10. Talano, J. F., Scanlon, P. J., Khan, M., Meadows, W. R., Loeb, H. S., Pifarre, R., and Gunnar, R. 1974. Influence of surgery on survival in 145 patients with LMCA disease. Circulation 49–50 (Suppl. III): III-110. (Abstr.).
11. Oliva, P. B., Potts, D. E., and Pluss, R. G. 1973. Coronary arterial spasm in Prinzmetal angina: documentation by coronary arteriography. New Engl. J. Med. 288: 745.
12. McAlpin, R. N., Kattus, A. A., and Alvaro, A. B. 1973. Angina pectoris at rest with preservation of exercise capacity. Circulation 47: 946.
13. Bulkley, B. H. and Roberts, W. C. 1974. Severe narrowing of LMCA: an indication of generalized severe coronary atherosclerosis. Circulation 49–50 (Suppl. III): III-150. (Abstr.).

# 4
# Unstable Angina Pectoris

L. Resnekov, M.D., J. Al-Sadir, M.D.,
R. E. Falicov, M.D. and C. E. Anagnostopoulos, M.D.

The epidemic of coronary heart disease continues unabated. It has been estimated that in this country more than five million people between 40 and 50 years old suffer obstructive coronary arterial disease (1). Each year more than 600,000 die as a result of the ailment, and close to 1 million persons are disabled. There are probably 150 to 200 thousand new cases of angina pectoris diagnosed each year (2) and the enormous proportions of the problem presented by these figures can hardly be overestimated. Further review of these facts reveals that 50% or more of deaths due to acute myocardial infarction occur within the first hour of the onset of symptoms, yet 70% of those dying do so before being brought to hospital. Although some 50% of patients who have suffered acute myocardial infarction report symptoms during the previous 2 to 3 months, suggesting that a dramatic change in their health has occurred, it is not true that 50% of patients with angina pectoris must inevitably develop myocardial infarction. It is clear, however, that the mortality of coronary heart disease could be dramatically reduced by the early identification and treatment of people at risk of developing myocardial infarction.

Recently there has been an introduction of myocardial revascularization surgery by direct coronary arterial bypass procedures using either the saphenous vein (3, 4) or the internal mammary artery (5, 6) for an anastomosis between the ascending aorta and the coronary artery or arteries beyond the obstruction. Such surgery offers the possibility of preventing myocardial infarction provided the population at risk can be identified. Unfortunately, although accepted as a concept by many, there is no definite evidence at the present time that surgical treatment is more

Supported by United States Public Health Service Contract NO1 HV-81334 Myocardial Infarction Research Unit.

effective than medical therapy in impending infarction and, furthermore, the incidence of infarction which may follow coronary arterial bypass surgery for stable angina pectoris is as high as 21% (7). The relative merit of medical versus surgical therapy in unstable angina pectoris both in the short- and long-term follow-up is as yet undetermined.

## CLINICAL SPECTRUM

Unstable angina pectoris can be defined as a changing situation presenting in one of several ways: 1) recent onset of angina pectoris, 2) changing pattern of angina pectoris, 3) angina pectoris occurring at rest. These three sub-groups frequently coexist. Furthermore, the pain characteristics can be subdivided into episodes of discrete attacks of pain, several discrete episodes or multiple daily episodes of pain. Similarly, the patients may be divided into those who have had previous stable angina pectoris, those with no previous episodes of cardiac pain, and those who have or have not had previous myocardial infarction.

Transient S-T and/or T wave changes may frequently occur and a shift in the S-T segment of at least 1 to 2 mm. upwards or downwards with or without associated T wave changes is often recorded during the attack of pain. Once the pain has subsided it is very common for the ECG record to return to the control state (Fig. 1).

To avoid confusion it is important whenever a diagnosis of unstable angina pectoris is being considered carefully to exclude myocardial infarc-

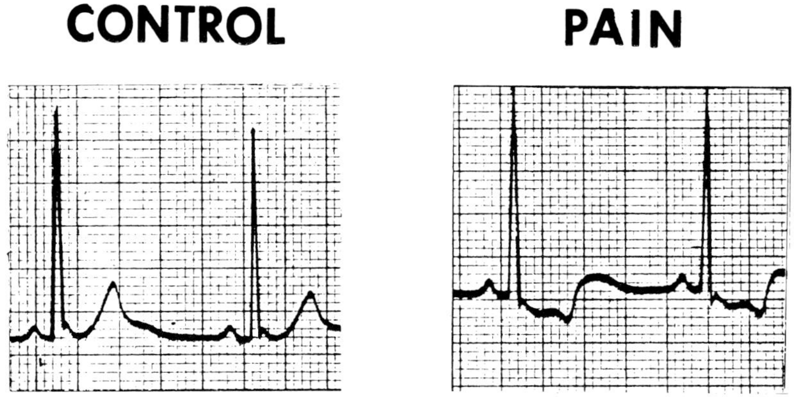


Figure 1. Electrocardiogram in unstable angina pectoris. Diagnostic S-T segment depression is recorded during cardiac pain but the tracing returns to the control record once pain has ceased.

tion. The appearance of new or persistent Q waves during the period following admission to hospital and any diagnostic elevation of the serum enzymes CPK, SGOT, SGPT, and LDH repeated serially would indicate that infarction has occurred and negate a diagnosis of unstable angina pectoris.

These clinical criteria describe, therefore, a patient with one or more attacks of severe cardiac pain associated with S-T and T wave changes but without the appearance of Q waves or a rise in serum enzyme levels consistent with a diagnosis of myocardial infarction.

## CLINICAL COURSE AND MANAGEMENT

The management of unstable angina pectoris remains both a therapeutic challenge and dilemma, for there is as yet no clear cut evidence regarding the effectiveness of medical or surgical therapy either in the short or long term. Nor are there yet data to advise an optimal time for coronary bypass surgery should the physician recommend surgical intervention.

Once acute myocardial infarction has been excluded and a diagnosis of unstable angina pectoris arrived at, it would seem highly desirable to assess the nature and extent of any coronary arterial obstructive lesions present so that a decision about possible surgery can be taken on firm anatomical grounds. Selective coronary arteriography should be performed using the Judkins or Sones technique with sufficient selective injections of the right and left coronary arteries made in various projections so that a detailed coronary anatomical profile can be arrived at. At the same time left ventricular function should be assessed by selectively injecting contrast material into that chamber and performing ciné-ventriculography, preferably in two planes. From these, end systolic and diastolic volumes and the ejection fraction can be derived and any associated lesions, for example mitral regurgitation, ventricular akinesis, dyskinesis, or aneurysm recognized.

Patients with unstable angina pectoris require intensive medical management preferably in a coronary care unit where their course can be carefully monitored. Treatment should include bedrest, oxygen, beta adrenergic blocking drugs, long acting nitrates, nitrites, analgesia, sedation, and digitalis and diuretic therapy when indicated. Many physicians use anticoagulant therapy, particularly with heparin although there are little data available to support its efficacy.

Continuing pain despite vigorous medical therapy indicates the need for considering surgical treatment. Similarly, younger patients, those whose electrocardiograms show the most marked S-T segment deviations and those with severely obstructed proximal portions of the coronary arteries, particularly the left main and the left anterior descending arteries, may require early surgery. In contrast, a prompt response to medical therapy and continued freedom from pain, absence of rhythm disturbances and a generally uncomplicated course might suggest continued medical therapy, including careful follow-up at 3-monthly intervals once discharged from hospital, to determine further management and the need for surgical intervention later on.

## DISCUSSION

For many years it has been recognized that the classical syndrome of angina pectoris has many variations, including the type, severity, and frequency of the associated chest pain as well as the ECG patterns recorded with the symptoms. Prinzmetal and his colleagues (8, 9) presumed that increased vascular tone in a vessel with obstructive lesions could lead transiently to a critically diminished blood supply to the area of the myocardium supplied, thus stimulating interest in an unusual clinical presentation. Variations in angina pectoris, however, were well recognized by many authorities several decades earlier (10–15), although the natural history of the untreated condition has not been fully established even up to the present time. Furthermore, the differences in definition and methods of management in reported series (16–22) make comparison extremely difficult if not impossible. Table I lists the terminology frequently used in the literature to describe clinical conditions suggestive of "unstable angina pectoris." As will be appreciated, these are frequently based on unproven assumptions regarding prognosis and pathophysiology, or on special groupings and clinical descriptors.

A prospective study of unstable angina pectoris (Table II) conducted by Fulton et al. (23) of the University of Edinburgh reported that among 230 patients, of whom 121 had recent angina pectoris, 92 changing patterns of angina pectoris, and 17 a recurrence of angina pectoris, the overall incidence of sudden death was 2% and of definite or suspected myocardial infarction 12.6%. Thus, the total complication rate for infarction or sudden death was about 15%, nor did this vary in the three groups of patients presenting with unstable angina pectoris. On the other hand, others report mortality figures which vary from 3 to 40% (20–22, 24, 25).

In addition, further confusion is provided by conflicting reports of surgical experience. Thus, Krauss et al. (26) documented an 86% survival at 1 year in a medically treated series of 104 patients but five deaths in a series of 32 patients treated surgically (27). This is in contrast to a

Table I. Terminology

| Terminology | Comments |
|---|---|
| Pre-infarction<br>Impending infarction | Based on:<br>Presumed prognosis |
| Variant angina pectoris<br>Prinzmetal angina pectoris<br>Status anginosus | Based on:<br>Special grouping |
| Acute coronary insufficiency<br>Coronary failure<br>Slight coronary attack | Based on:<br>Presumed pathophysiology |
| Unstable angina pectoris<br>Intermediate syndrome<br>Crescendo angina<br>Rest angina<br>Angina decubitus<br>Nocturnal angina | Based on:<br>Clinical descriptor |

mortality of 5% at the same institution for an identical operation on patients with *stable* angina pectoris. Others, however, report a surgical mortality for "pre-infarction" patients of 5% or less (28), yet a mortality varying from 7 to 22% is reported among 145 patients operated on for unstable angina pectoris in four separate series (29–32). There is, therefore, a wide range of surgical mortality in the group of patients with unstable angina pectoris but a relatively constant mortality of 5% or less for the same operation performed by the same surgical team when angina pectoris is stable.

Experience with stable angina pectoris indicates that estimates of mortality based on the coronary arteriographic anatomy are far more precise than those based on the clinical definition alone (33). For this reason we are recommending coronary arteriographic characterization in all patients in whom the diagnosis of unstable angina pectoris has been made and acute myocardial infarction excluded.

The late follow-up of these patients is similarly not yet established. In an important study by Gazes et al. (34) there was a cumulative survival rate among 140 patients of 82% at 12 months, 75% at 24 months, 69% at 36 months, 61% at 60 months, and 48% at 10 years. Twenty-one percent of these patients developed acute myocardial infarction within 8 months of diagnosis of unstable angina pectoris, in whom there was a mortality of 41%. Useful as this information undoubtedly is, no information is available

Table II. Unstable Angina Pectoris Prospective Trial, Edinburgh Series[a]

| Presentation | No. | Sudden Death | Acute M.I. Definite or Suspected | Cardiac Arrest | Total |
|---|---|---|---|---|---|
| Recent angina | 121 | 2 | 16 | 0 | 18 (15%) |
| Changing angina | 92 | 3 | 10 | 1 | 14 (15%) |
| Recurrent angina | 17 | 0 | 0 | 0 | 3 (18%) |
| Total | 230 | 5 (2%) | 29 (12.6%) | 1 | 35 (15.2%) |

[a]Modified from Fulton et al. (23).

regarding the coronary anatomy of these patients and the extent or even presence of any coronary arterial obstructive disease.

Factors which appear to worsen the prognosis of unstable angina pectoris are as follows:

1. Clinical: Persistent pain despite vigorous therapy, recurrent rhythm disturbances, and the development of congestive cardiac failure.
2. Electrocardiographic: Florid S-T segment shift or T wave changes during pain.
3. Hemodynamics: Poor left ventricular function.
4. Coronary anatomy: Severity and extent of the lesions.

Several groups have reported the risks of undertaking selective coronary arteriography and left ventriculography in patients with unstable angina pectoris. Thus, Conti et al. (32) had one death during angiography and another shortly thereafter among 57 consecutive patients being studied. Scanlon et al. (35) reported that cardiac catheterization and angiography were performed without major complications in 97% of 85 patients. More recently, Loop and others (36) have confirmed that these investigations can be undertaken in this unstable group of patients without a significantly increased risk as compared to patients with stable angina pectoris.

Unstable angina pectoris appears to be a disease particularly affecting the left coronary arterial system and severe obstructive lesions of the proximal portions of the left anterior descending and circumflex arteries are common. Since left main coronary arterial obstruction is also frequently found in this group of patients its exclusion by selective coronary arteriography is a further argument in favor of undertaking cardiac catheterization studies as a routine once the diagnosis of unstable angina pectoris has been made. It is well recognized that coronary arterial spasm may be demonstrated in patients with this clinical syndrome in the absence of fixed obstructive lesions and a significant number of patients may have no important epicardial coronary arterial disease (35).

The so-called Prinzmetal angina (8, 9) has rightfully been considered unstable and a very high mortality reported (38). More recently, however, (38–42) it has been determined that also in Prinzmetal angina there is a wide spectrum of coronary arterial abnormality varying from spasm to fixed obstruction in one and frequently in several of the coronary arteries. The expected prognosis is now known to be better than originally feared, a mortality of 5% in the first 3 months being reported (38). Response to medical therapy is often good and may even be better than surgical treatment. Gaasch and his group (43) reported that only 38% of 24 patients operated on were free of pain and that 29% had no symptomatic improvement whatsoever. Their in-hospital surgical mortality was 12%.

The occurence of pain in association with S-T segment shift is widely used in the diagnosis of unstable angina pectoris. It is now clear that episodic S-T segment change can be recorded by tape monitoring patients either at bedrest or when up and about in the complete absence of any chest pain (44). In these patients too, important occlusive disease of the coronary arteries can be demonstrated by selective coronary arteriography. The natural history of this painless form of episodic S-T segment depression is as yet unknown.

Follow-up studies once the patient has been discharged from the hospital indicate that the incidence of myocardial infarction is higher in patients treated surgically but that by and large medically treated patients have a higher incidence of angina pectoris and live more restricted lives (32, 35).

A randomized trial comparing the results in the short and long term of medical and surgical management of unstable angina pectoris is badly needed to provide guidance for the appropriate treatment of this group of patients. Such a trial is at present being conducted under the auspices of the National Institutes of Health through its Myocardial Infarction Research Unit program and preliminary results (45) have now been published on 138 patients, 73 of whom received medical and 65 surgical therapy. There were four surgical and two medical in-hospital deaths and after a mean follow-up of 7 months two further surgical group and three further medical group deaths occurred. Fourteen of the surgical patients developed myocardial infarction in-hospital and in this group five late myocardial infarctions occurred. There were fewer myocardial infarctions in the medical group, six during the in-hospital phase and five later on but the medical patients had a far higher incidence of angina pectoris. No firm conclusions can yet be drawn from this study and the results of further patients randomized to medical or surgical therapy is needed and particularly the results of the late follow-up.

Unstable angina pectoris is likely to be due to a sudden change in myocardial perfusion in patients with already well developed coronary atherosclerotic lesions. These commonly present as high grade obstructions of the left anterior descending and circumflex arteries, particularly in their proximal portions. Obstruction of the left main coronary artery is relatively frequent. The coronary anatomy differs, therefore, very little from that demonstrated in patients with other forms of coronary heart disease. The major complication of unstable angina pectoris is the development of acute myocardial infarction and, fortunately, sudden death is less common. Overall ventricular function is similar to that in any other form of coronary heart disease and depends on the severity and extent of the coronary arterial lesion, the previous incidence of infarction, and the development of an adequate collateral circulation, varying from slight alteration to severe dysfunction. The overall prognosis can be related in part to the degree of abnormality present. Since the coronary anatomical lesions and their effects on the heart are so similar to that found in stable angina pectoris, what additional abnormality results in the condition becoming unstable? It is likely that the clinical syndrome is produced by a sudden physiological change when coronary obstructive lesions are developed to a critical extent and that abrupt demands in myocardial oxygen consumption relative to the supply available result in the clinical picture. This view is supported by Lambert et al. (46).

Although it is still premature to advocate the superiority of medical or surgical therapy during the acute phase of the syndrome it is appropriate to offer the following guidelines for patient management once the diagnosis of unstable angina pectoris has been made. Medical treatment, if decided upon, should be undertaken in a coronary care unit where patients can be carefully monitored and their course observed. The aims of such treatment are first to reduce myocardial oxygen consumption and second to increase the available oxygen supply to the heart muscle. As such, beta adrenergic blocking drugs and sedation can be used to reduce both heart rate and contractility. Any associated systemic hypertension and any increase in heart size should be treated by appropriate therapy to reduce myocardial wall stress. In an attempt to increase the available oxygen supply and thereby to limit myocardial ischemia and to prevent infarction, nitrites and oxygen can be recommended. Surgical treatment, on the other hand, would be recommended as an acute intervention in an attempt to increase significantly myocardial perfusion, thereby limiting the size of the ischemic zone by revascularizing the surrounding area. Additional benefits could be the prevention of serious ventricular dysfunction and abolishing or preventing recurrent ventricular rhythm disturbances.

The preliminary results of the randomized trial (45) suggest that there is an equal mortality but a higher myocardial infarction rate in the surgically treated group and that the incidence of angina pectoris in follow-up is greater in the medical group. Final conclusions however must await the results of studying further patients and a longer period of follow-up.

## SUMMARY

The clinical spectrum of unstable angina pectoris is reviewed and guidelines offered for patient management. Patients with unstable angina pectoris should be treated initially in a coronary care unit and myocardial infarction excluded by serial electrocardiograms and serum enzyme determinations. Medical therapy should be given with vigor, including: bed-rest, sedation, oxygen, beta adrenergic blockade, nitrites, and long acting nitrates. Any associated hypertension, anemia, or thyrotoxicosis should be treated. The majority of patients will respond to this form of therapy and will become pain-free. The major complication of the syndrome is acute myocardial infarction (13%), whereas sudden death is fortunately less common (3%). The coronary anatomical lesion(s) should be determined by selective arteriography as soon as acute myocardial infarction has been excluded and at the same time ventricular function should be assessed and any associated conditions excluded, such as mitral regurgitation, ventricular aneurysm, or dyskinetic or akinetic segments. Patients with high grade proximal obstructive lesions, those with obstructions to the left main coronary artery, and those who persist with cardiac pain should be considered for early coronary bypass surgery. It is still unclear whether in the short or long term medical or surgical therapy is superior, but preliminary results from an ongoing randomized trial suggest an equal mortality but a higher incidence of myocardial infarction in the surgical group. Continuing angina pectoris is more frequent when patients are treated medically. Those with so-called Prinzmetal angina should be considered as having unstable angina pectoris and managed according to the principles outlined above.

## REFERENCES

1. Mullins, C. B. 1973. Evaluation of coronary artery surgery—one step forward. Ann. Intern. Med. 78: 447.

2. Glenn, W. W. L. 1972. Some reflections on the coronary bypass operation. Circulation 45: 869.
3. Favoloro, R. G. 1968. Saphenous vein autograft replacement of severe segmental coronary artery occlusion. Operation technique. Ann. Thorac. Surg. 5: 334.
4. Johnson, W. D., Flemma, R. J., Lepley, D. Jr., et al. 1969. Extended treatment of severe coronary artery disease: a total surgical approach. Ann. Surg. 170: 460.
5. Kolessov, J. 1967. Mammary artery–coronary artery anastomosis as method of treatment for angina pectoris. J. Thorac. Cardiovasc. Surg. 54: 535.
6. Green, G. E., Spencer, F. C., Tice, D. A. et al. 1972. Arterial and venous microsurgical bypass grafts for coronary artery disease. J. Thorac. Cardiovasc. Surg. 14: 260.
7. Dunkman, W. B., Perloff, J. K., Kastor, J. A., and Shelburne, J. C. 1974. Medical perspectives in coronary artery surgery–a caveat. Ann. Intern. Med. 81: 817.
8. Prinzmetal, M., Kennamer, R., Merliss, R., Wada, T., and Bor, N. 1959. Angina pectoris I–A variant form of angina pectoris. Am. J. Med. 27: 35.
9. Prinzmetal, M. Ekmekci, A., Kennamer, R. Kwoczynski, J. K., Shubin, H., and Toyoshima, H. 1960. Variant form of angina pectoris. JAMA 174: 1794.
10. Hausner, E. and Sherf, D. 1933. Uber angina pectoris–Probleme. Z Klin Med. 126: 166.
11. Borw, G. R. and Holman, D. V. 1933. Electrocardiographic study during a paroxysm of angina pectoris. Am. Heart J. 9: 259.
12. Burrett, J. B. 1939. High take-off of the S-T segment without coronary occlusion. Bull N. Y. Med. Coll. 2: 121.
13. Wilson, F. N. and Johnston, F. D. 1941. The occurrence in angina pectoris of electrocardiographic changes similar in magnitude and in kind to those produced by myocardial infarction. Am. Heart J. 22: 64.
14. Sanazaro, P. J. 1956. Transient electrocardiographic changes simulating myocardial infarction. Am. Heart J. 51: 149.
15. Parkinson, J. and Bedford, E. 1931. Electrocardiographic changes during brief attacks of angina pectoris. Lancet 1: 15.
16. Owren, P. A. 1963. Coronary artery insufficiency. Dis. Chest 44: 561.
17. Papp, C. and Smith, K. S. 1960. Status anginosus. Br. Heart J. 22: 259.
18. Vakil, R. J. 1961. Intermediate coronary syndrome. Circulation 24: 557.
19. Mounsey, P. 1951. Prodromal symptoms in myocardial infarction. Br. Heart J. 13: 215.
20. Wood, P. 1961. Acute and subacute coronary insufficiency. Br. Med. J. 1: 1779.
21. Resnik, W. H. 1962. Pre-infarction angina. II. An interpretation. Mod. Conc. Cardiovasc. Dis. 31: 757.
22. Levy, H. 1956. The natural history of changing patterns of angina pectoris. Ann. Intern. Med. 44: 1123.

23. Fulton, M., Duncan, B., Lutz, W., Morrison, S. L., Donald, K. W., Kerr, F., Kirby, B. J., Julian, D. G., and Oliver, M. R. 1972. Natural history of unstable angina. Lancet 1: 860.
24. Vakil, R. J. 1964. Pre-Infarction syndrome—Management and follow-up. Am. J. Cardiol. 14: 55.
25. Resnik, W. H. 1962. The significance of prolonged anginal pain (pre-infarction angina). Am. Heart J. 63: 290.
26. Krauss, K. R., Hutter, A. M., and DeSanctis, R. W. 1972. Acute coronary insufficiency: Course and follow-up. Arch. Intern. Med. 129: 808.
27. Conti, C. R., Greene, B., Pitt, B., Griffith, L., Humphries, O. N., Brawley, R., Taylor, D., Bender, H., Gott, V., and Ross, R. S. 1971. Coronary surgery in unstable angina pectoris. Circulation 44: 154.
28. Auer, J. E., Johnson, W. D. Flemma, R. J., Tector, A. J., and Lepley, D. Jr. 1971. Direct coronary artery surgery for impending myocardial infarction. Circulation 44: 102. (Abstr.).
29. Fischl, S. J., Herman, M. V., and Gorlin, R. 1973. The intermediate coronary syndrome. Clinical, angiographic and therapeutic aspects. N. Engl. J. Med. 288: 1193.
30. Bertolasi, C. A., Tronge, J. E., Capreno, C. A. et al. 1974. Unstable angina. Prospective and randomized study of its evaluation, with and without surgery. Am. J. Cardiol. 33: 201.
31. Miller, D. C., Cannom, D. S., Fogarty, T. J. et al. 1973. Saphenous vein coronary artery bypass in patients with "pre-infarction angina." Circulation 47: 234.
32. Conti, C. R., Brawley, R. K., Griffith, L. S. C., Pitt, B., Humphries, J. W., Gott, V. L., and Ross, R. S. 1973. Unstable angina pectoris: Morbidity and mortality in 57 consecutive patients evaluated angiographically. Am. J. Cardiol., 32: 745.
33. Friesinger, G. C., Page, E. E., and Ross, R. S. 1970. Prognostic significance of coronary arteriography. Trans. Assoc. Am. Phys. 83: 78.
34. Gazes, P. C., Mobley, E. M., Jr., Faris, H. M., Jr., Duncan, R. S., and Humphries, G. B. 1973. Pre-infarctional (unstable) angina—a prospective—ten-year follow-up. Circulation 48: 331.
35. Scanlon, P. J., Nemickas, R., Moran J. F., Talano, J. V., Amirparviz, F., and Pifarré, R. Accelerated angina pectoris—Clinical, hemodynamic, arteriographic and therapeutic experience in 85 patients. Circulation 47: 19.
36. Loop, F. D., Cheanvechai, C., Sheldon, W. C., Taylor, P. C., and Effler, D. B. 1974. Early myocardial revascularization during acute myocardial infarction. Chest 66: 478.
37. Silverman, M. E. and Flamm, M. D., Jr: Variant angina pectoris. Anatomic findings and prognostic implications. Ann. Intern. Med. 75: 339.
38. McAlpin, R. N., Kattus, A. A., and Alvaro, A. B. 1973. Angina pectoris at rest with preservation of exercise capacity. Prinzmetal's variant angina. Circulation 47: 946.
39. Dhurandhar, R. W., Watt, D. L., Silver, M. D., et al. 1972. Prinzmetal's variant form of angina with arteriographic evidence of coronary arterial spasm. Am. J. Cardiol. 30: 902.

40. Cheng, T. O., Bashour, T., Kelser, G. A., Jr., et al. 1973. Variant angina of Prinzmetal with normal coronary arteriograms. A variant of the variant. Circulation 47: 476.
41. Bete, J. M., Shubrooks, S. J., Block, P. C., et al. 1973. Prinzmetal's angina pectoris, clinical and anatomical spectrum and results of coronary artery surgery (abstract). Circulation 48 (Suppl. IV): IV-145.
42. Ruggeroli, C. W., Cohn, K., and Langston, M. 1974. Prinzmetal's variant angina: a pathophysiological and clinical kaleidoscope (abstract). Am. J. Cardiol. 33: 167.
43. Gassch, W. H., Lufschanowski, R., Leachman, R. D., and Alexander, J. K. 1974. Surgical management of Prinzmetal's variant angina. Chest 66: 614.
44. Kossowsky, W. A., Mohr, B. D., Summers, D. M., and Lyon, A. F. 1974. Further variant patterns within Prinzmetal angina pectoris. Chest 66: 622.
45. Conti, C. R., Gilbert, J. B., Hodget, M., Hutter, A. N., Jr., Kaplan, E. N., Newell, J. B., Resnekov, L., Rosati, R. A., Ross, R. S., Russell, R. O., Jr., Schroeder, J. S., and Wolk, M. 1975. Unstable angina pectoris: Randomized study of surgical versus medical therapy. Am. J. Cardiol. 35: 28.
46. Lambert, C. J., Adam, M., and Geisler, G. F. 1971. Emergency myocardial revascularization for impending infarctions and arrhythmias. J. Thorac. Cardiovasc. Surg. 62: 522.

# 5 Panel on Coronary Disease

**Moderator**
L. Resnekov, M.D.
**Panel Members**
R. M. Gunnar, M.D., R. E. Falicov, M.D.,
J. M. Moran, M.D., J. J. Lamberti, M.D. and C. E. Anagnostopoulos, M.D.

**Dr. Resnekov**: The coronary anatomy in unstable angina appears to be similar to that seen in stable angina. Why, therefore, does a patient become unstable at a particular time? What is the pathophysiology of the syndrome?

**Dr. Gunnar**: It is not clear why patients become unstable at a particular time in the course of the disease. However, it is to be stressed that in patients with main left coronary artery obstructions, whether angina is accelerating or not, a high mortality is seen. Perhaps, if huge numbers of patients were studied, it could be shown that the patients with an unstable pattern of symptoms carry a higher mortality, but at present the difference between these patients and those with stable angina does not appear to be great. Unstable angina has been defined as an angina with an accelerating pattern over a short period of time to the point where the patient is incapacitated and where myocardial infarction is thought to be impending.

**Dr. Falicov**: The coronary arteriogram gives us only an anatomical description of the lesions present but we cannot directly predict from the pictures the clinical symptoms or their progressions. For example in an 80% obstruction of a coronary artery, a very small increase in the severity of the obstruction may result in a significant decrease in blood flow and lead to accelerated symptoms.

**Dr. Resnekov:** We have heard today that main left coronary obstruction is a devastating disease. If diagnosed, therefore, at what point should surgery be undertaken to prevent the risk of death? Is this disease a surgical emergency, Dr. Lamberti?

**Dr. Lamberti:** Catheterization of main left lesions has been said to have a higher risk, and the clinical course after catheterization appears to be accelerated. Patients with significant stenosis of the left main coronary artery often require urgent intervention. If the patient experiences chest pain in the catheterization laboratory or afterwards, he is taken directly to the operating room for revascularization. If the patient is stable following study, we have occasionally used tight medical management and pursued a course of early, elective operation. Generally, we have revascularized significant left main coronary artery stenosis within 24 hr. after diagnosis. In spite of emergency surgery, an operative mortality greater than that seen in other types of coronary disease has been reported. For chronic stable angina, operative mortality less than 2% should be obtained, whereas for left main coronary disease, an 8 to 10% operative mortality has been reported by others. At this institution, patients with main left coronary lesions are occasionally sedated and operated on more than 24 hr. after catheterization without apparent risk. However, we are always prepared to operate as soon as possible if necessary. We have not seen an increased surgical mortality in patients with left main stenosis operated on at the University of Chicago.

**Dr. Resnekov:** Summarizing your position on this issue, Dr. Lamberti, left main coronary lesions without continuing cardiac pain should be dealt with as a relative surgical emergency. If there is cardiac pain revascularization surgery should be done without delay as an emergency. Dr. Moran, would you comment?

**Dr. Moran:** I agree with Dr. Lamberti. Our experience at Loyola University has been similar. We have often been surprised to find at surgery a bluish myocardium with a paradoxically moving left ventricle even when this had not been suspected earlier. These patients may become unstable quite unpredictably, indicating that oxygen supply to the myocardium is in a precarious state.

**Dr. Resnekov:** The results of surgery appear to depend in large part in patency of the graft. Dr. Anagnostopoulos, what factors are important in assuring long-term patency?

**Dr. Anagnostopoulos:** It is important not to allow the graft to twist at the time of operation and in addition to perfect technique in the anastomosis, it would be ideal if one could perform angiography in the operating room. This at present is not feasible but it is an accepted procedure to measure the coronary flow at the time of operation. It has been shown that the likelihood of graft occlusion is increased if the flow is under 40 ml/min.

**Dr. Resnekov:** Do anticoagulants affect graft patency?

**Dr. Lamberti:** There is no really solid evidence that anticoagulation plays a role in the management of postoperative coronary bypass patients. Some have used anticoagulation following endarterectomy of the right coronary artery. Barner, in St. Louis, utilized this exclusively for internal mammary bypass graft with endarterectomy of the right coronary arter and he reported a 90% patency rate at 1 year. This represents the highest patency reported in the management of such lesions. Of course, in lesions of the anterior descending coronary artery, internal mammary artery grafts have been shown to have superior patency rates over the long term.

**Dr. Resnekov:** Dr. Falicov, would you summarize the indications for coronary arteriography?

**Dr. Falicov:** A history of angina pectoris, or the development of a highly positive exercise test are certainly the main indications for angiography. A number of patients also undergo study because of chest pain of uncertain cause. The procedure is the best means of diagnosing coronary arterial disease and can be done swiftly with a very low morbidity and mortality.

**Dr. Anagnostopoulos:** In the University of Chicago series of over 500 patients, there have been no deaths or serious complications due to coronary angiography. About 35 of the patients in this series had unstable angina or main left coronary artery lesions. None died following scheduled surgery.

**Dr. Resnekov:** Is there any difference in pain or mortality in patients in whom the graft remains patent as compared to those in whom the graft occludes?

**Dr. Lamberti:** For the most part, patients who are pain-free have patent grafts. However, a small number of patients with occluded grafts are pain-free. This may be explained by infarction of the area of the myocardium which produced the pain. Generally if one looks at the group of patients undergoing coronary surgery, about 80% are symptom-free or are markedly improved.

**Question from the floor**: Is the internal mammary artery still being implanted into the myocardium for coronary disease?

**Dr. Moran**: This procedure, called the Vineberg operation, has largely gone out of vogue in this country, but it may have had a premature death. There are cases in which impressive collaterals developed after the implantation.

**Question from the floor**: If an artery is totally occluded and the patient is symptomatic is such an operation recommended?

**Dr. Lamberti**: We have sometimes found that when more than one vessel is involved a combination of surgical techniques may be used. For example, a vein bypass graft may be used for the left anterior descending artery, and if the circumflex is totally occluded for much of its length or is inoperable by virtue of its anatomical location within the myocardium, or if much disease is present distally, the internal mammary artery may be mobilized and implanted into the posterior portion of the left ventricle.

**Dr. Anagnostopoulos**: Under no circumstances should both vein grafting and internal artery implantation by undertaken to the same area of myocardium. The stimulus to collateral vessels in the mammary implant is anoxia and if an area is directly perfused by blood from a vein graft there is no reason to do both procedures.

**Dr. Gunnar**: I would like to stress that the intra-aortic balloon finds application in many of the patients discussed earlier. It alleviates pain and often stabilizes the patients hemodynamically until surgery.

**Dr. Resnekov**: Thank you.

# Transposition II

Complete Transposition
of the Great Arteries
Physiology, Diagnosis
and Medical Management

Surgical Treatment
of Transposition
of the Great Arteries:
Technical Considerations
and Results

Panel on
Transposition

# 6 Complete Transposition of the Great Arteries: Physiology, Diagnosis, and Medical Management

R. A. Arcilla, M.D.

Transposition of the great arteries is one of the common types of congenital heart disease. It accounts for approximately 15% of all congenital cardiac diseases encountered in the neonatal period (1, 2), and has been estimated to occur once in every 3000 to 4500 births (3, 4).

The anomaly may occur in several types, depending on the position of the great arteries and their ventricles of origin. The most common type, ordinarily referred to as d-transposition (simple or non-inverted transposition), occurs in approximately 70% of all transposition complexes. It is characterized by reversal of the anteroposterior relationship of the aorta and pulmonary artery to each other, and by reversal of their ventricles of origin. The aorta arises from the right ventricle, and the pulmonary artery from the left ventricle. In the normally-positioned heart (levocardia), the aorta lies anteriorly and often to the right of the pulmonary trunk; in the rare cases with mirror-image dextrocardia, it lies anteriorly and usually to the left of the pulmonary trunk. D-transposition is also ordinarily known

Supported in part by a grant (RR-305) from the General Clinical Research Centers Program Division of Research Resources, National Institutes of Health.

by the general or nondescript term, complete transposition of the great arteries (CTGA). This paper is devoted to a discussion of this form of transposition.

Other types of transposition complexes include single ventricle with transposition of the great arteries (14%), double-outlet right ventricle (10%), where both vessels arise from the right ventricle, and inverted or l-transposition of the great arteries (6%). The latter is usually accompanied by atrioventricular discordance, i.e., the right atrium opens into the anatomic left ventricle whereas the left atrium opens into the anatomic right ventricle. The aorta which arises from the latter chamber is to the left of, and somewhat anterior to the pulmonary trunk. This complex is also ordinarily referred to by the nondescript term, corrected transposition of the great vessels.

The hemodynamics, clinical features, and management of CTGA are influenced by the presence or absence of significant ventricular septal defect or pulmonary stenosis. Accordingly, the anomaly is classified into:

I. CTGA with intact ventricular septum (IVS)
   A. Without pulmonary stenosis, 50%
   B. With pulmonary stenosis, 5%
II. CTGA with ventricular septal defect (VSD)
   A. Without pulmonary stenosis, 30%
   B. With pulmonary stenosis, 15%

The cases with small or restrictive VSD appropriately belong to the group of CTGA with IVS since the septal defect is not large enough to promote free shunting of blood and equalization of both ventricular pressures. On the other hand, those with pulmonary stenosis, even though mild, are classified in the pulmonary stenosis group since there is evidence that the left ventricular outflow obstruction, which is usually subvalvar but occasionally valvar or annular as well, tends to increase with age.

## PATHOPHYSIOLOGY

The normal fetal circulation is characterized, among other things, by the two ventricles functionally in parallel and equally maintaining the systemic circulation. Thus, whether the great vessels are in normal position or are transposed does not appear to be critical. After birth, however, after the establishment of the pulmonary circulation separately from the systemic circulation, the circulatory pattern in CTGA is immediately life threatening. The poorly oxygenated blood recirculates through the systemic circuit, whereas the highly oxygenated blood remains in the pulmonary circuit. For life to be possible, there must be adequate exchange between the two circuits (Fig. 1). This intercirculatory mixing site(s) may be at the atrial level (patent forament ovale or atrial septal defect), at the ventricular level (VSD), or at the level of the great vessels (patent ductus arteriosus or bronchial arteries). In CTGA with IVS, shunting across the atrial septal defect is predominantly from left atrium to right atrium during ventricular systole (due to the lower left atrial compliance), but is chiefly from right atrium to left atrium during ventricular diastole (due to the lower right ventricular than left ventricular compliance). Since the pulmonary artery pressure is much lower than that of the aorta, flow across an associated patent ductus arteriosus or across the bronchial arteries is chiefly from aorta to pulmonary artery.

In CTGA with VSD of significant size, shunting across the latter is bidirectional, presumably occurring during both phases of the cardiac

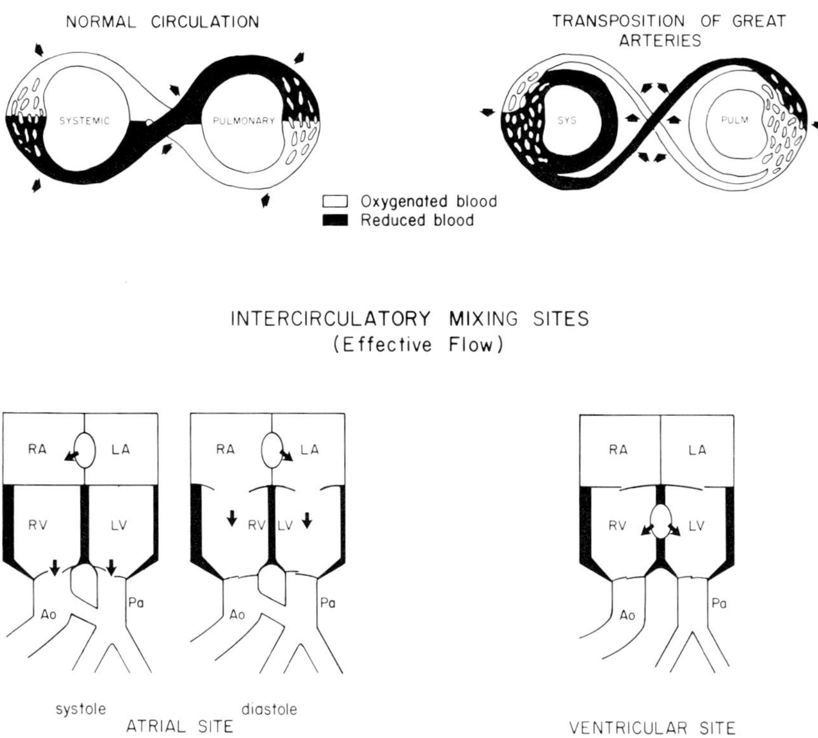


Figure 1. Schematic diagram of the normal circulation and of the circulation in complete transposition of the great vessels. Intercirculatory mixing (effective pulmonary blood flow) is shown by the blood columns from the two circuits which cross each other. The rest of the blood recirculates in the systemic or pulmonary circulations.

cycle. The large VSD promotes equilibration of pressures in both ventricles so that left ventricular and pulmonary artery pressures (in the absence of pulmonary stenosis) approximate those of the right ventricle and aorta. Over any sustained period of time, and irrespective of the shunting sites, the over-all right to left shunt equals that of the left to right shunt. The right to left shunt is also identified as the effective pulmonary blood flow (EPBF), i.e., that part of the systemic venous return which reaches the pulmonary vascular bed for gas exchange.

The degree of intercirculatory mixing depends on the number, size, and position of the above shunting defects or communications. It is, to a large extent, responsible for the systemic arterial oxygen saturation and the resultant $pO_2$ at which oxygen is delivered to the tissues. Generally speaking, positive correlation exists between the degree of intercirculatory mixing (synonymous with effective pulmonary blood flow) and total pulmonary blood flow (5). The latter is the sum of effective pulmonary flow and recirculating pulmonary flow. High systemic arterial oxygen saturation thus indicates not only good intercirculatory mixing but usually also increased total pulmonary flow, and vice versa. This generalization, however, is valid only when the mixing site(s) is adequate. In newborn infants with IVS, small or closing ductus and only a patent foramen ovale, there may be large total pulmonary flow with, however, only a small EPBF. The systemic arterial oxygen saturation in this instance is unusually low and often below 40%.

Whereas a large ventricular septal defect assures good intercirculatory mixing, it often results in too much pulmonary blood flow and severe heart failure early in infancy. In addition, the high pressures in the pulmonary circuit consequent to the VSD promote early and progressive pulmonary vascular changes which eventually result in pulmonary vascular obstruction (6, 7). A similar chain of events may result from a large patent ductus arteriosus with marked pulmonary hypertension. In CTGA with IVS, pulmonary vascular obstruction develops at a considerably slower pace, and is not a striking hemodynamic feature of the disease.

The pathophysiology in CTGA is briefly summarized in Figures 2 and 3. In the newborn period, the adequacy of intercirculatory mixing is critical. This is especially true in CTGA with IVS. Where the interatrial communication is a small defect or just a patent foramen ovale, there is not only marked systemic arterial oxygen desaturation but also, and paradoxically, increased pulmonary blood flow and pulmonary venous congestion. Pulmonary compliance is accordingly reduced. Early-onset heart failure also supervenes. During infancy and childhood, the sequelae of long standing hypoxemia become additional important features of the disease. There is an increase in red cell mass and in blood volume in

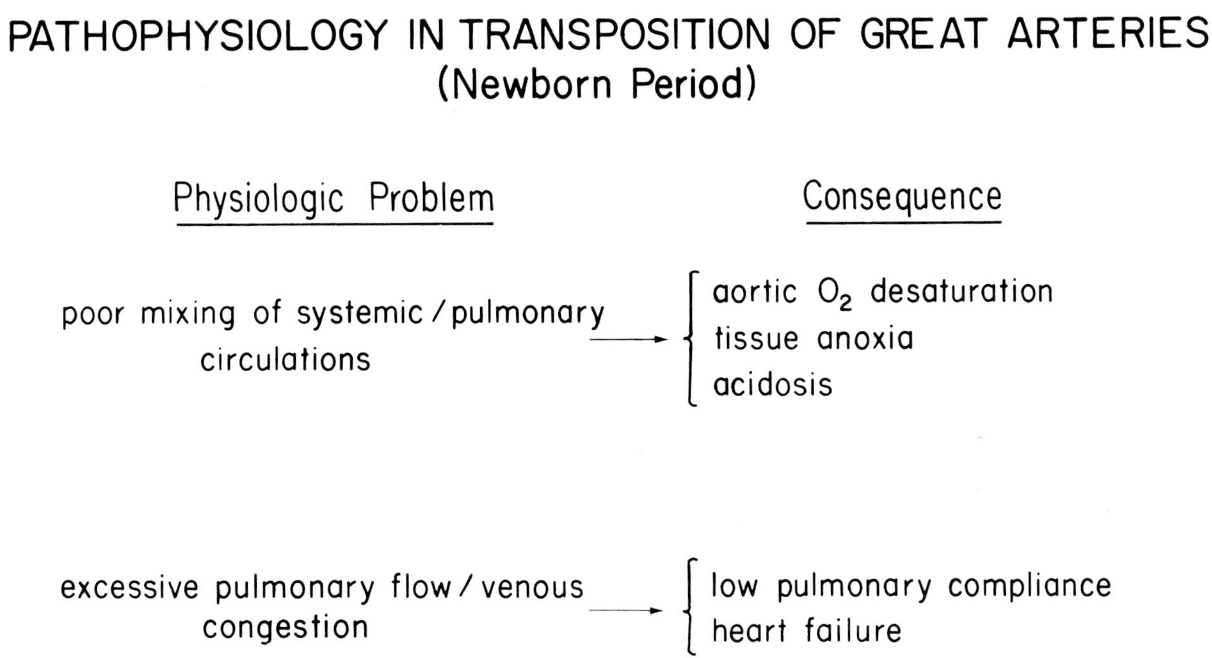


Figure 2. Pathophysiology of CTGA in newborn period.

PATHOPHYSIOLOGY IN TRANSPOSITION OF GREAT ARTERIES
(Infancy and Childhood)

| Physiologic Problem | | Consequence |
|---|---|---|
| inadequate mixing of systemic / pulmonary circulations | → | aortic $O_2$ desaturation<br>tissue hypoxia |
| secondary polycythemia | → | ↑ blood and red cell volume<br>↑ blood viscosity<br>↑ peripheral vascular resistance |
| cardiac overwork + low $O_2$ coronary perfusion | → | myocardial hypertrophy<br>myocardial fibrosis<br>myocardial failure |
| pulmonary vascular obstruction | → | irreversible pulmonary hypertension |

Figure 3. Pathophysiology of CTGA in infancy and childhood.

response to the decreased systemic arterial oxygen saturation. The polycythemia, when marked, results in significant increase in blood viscosity with corresponding alterations in the circulatory dynamics, e.g., increased peripheral vascular resistance, reduced cardiac output, increased shear stress, altered blood flow patterns, etc., which more than counterbalance the presumed benefit of an increase in oxygen carrying capacity of the hemoglobin-rich blood (8). Thromboembolic complications involving various organ systems or, more commonly, the central nervous system in the form of cerebrovascular accidents may also occur. In CTGA with VSD, pulmonary hypertension and progressing pulmonary vascular obstruction are additional pathophysiologic states of major therapeutic significance.

## DIAGNOSIS

The usual clinical manifestations are cyanosis at or shortly after birth, tachypnea, and heart failure of early onset. The typical newborn infant is a male (in about 65 to 75%) with normal gestational age and normal or increased birth weight. On examination, there is increased lower precordial movement due to right ventricular overwork, a single and loud second sound of aortic origin since pulmonic closure is often clinically inaudible, and a non-specific systolic murmur in about 80%. During the first 1 or 2 weeks of life there may be no murmur. In the presence of pulmonary stenosis, the murmur is louder, longer, and of typical ejection quality. In addition, it is frequently better heard over the right than left upper sternal border due to the abnormal trajectory of the pulmonary outflow tract which is directed towards the right base in this disease (Fig. 4). Breathlessness, frequent respiratory infections, and retarded physical growth and development are observed, together with the other usual signs of heart failure. After 4 to 6 months, the cyanosis is accompanied by clubbing of the digits, and by secondary polycythemia. The latter is manifested by increased venous hematocrit which shows positive correlation with systemic arterial oxygen saturation in cyanotic congenital heart disease after the age of 6 months (Fig. 5).

The chest roentgenograms during the 1st week may be within normal limits. Thereafter, progressive cardiomegaly involving most or all chambers is observed. An increase in pulmonary vascular markings is noted almost invariably in those without pulmonary stenosis. In the presence of the latter, cardiac enlargement is not as striking and involves chiefly the right ventricle; the pulmonary vascular markings also vary depending on the severity of the stenosis. Because of the abnormal position of the great vessels, with the pulmonary trunk lying almost directly behind the aorta,

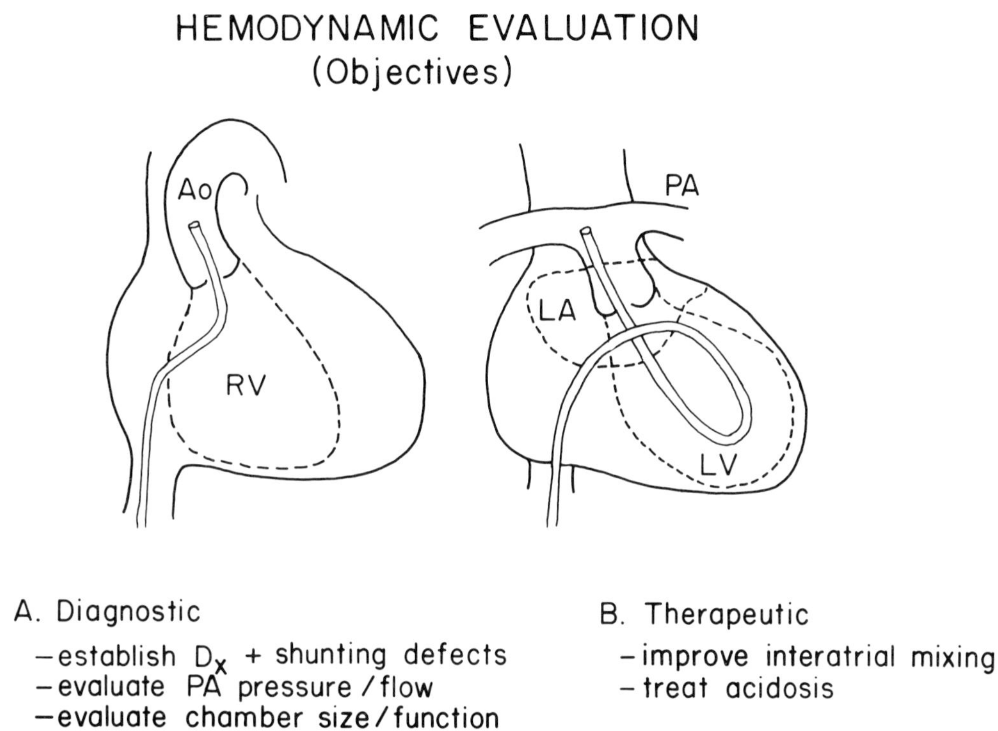


Figure 4. Positions of aortic catheter (from right ventricle) and of pulmonary artery catheter (from left ventricle) shown schematically in the frontal projection. The general objectives of the cardiac catheterization procedure are outlined.

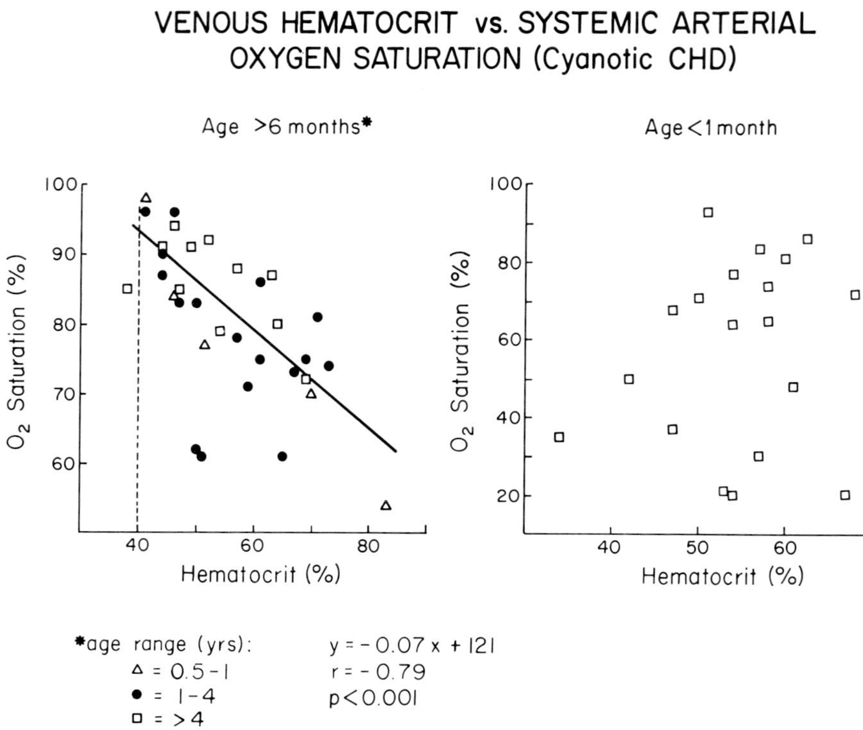


Figure 5. Systemic arterial oxygen saturation plotted against venous hematocrit in children 6 months of age or older (*left*) and in newborn infants (*right*). Vertical dotted line on left identifies the normal hematocrit level. Note positive correlation in the infants and children but absence of correlation in the neonates.

the vascular pedicle appears unusually narrow in about three-fourths of the cases (Fig. 6). The cardiac silhouette in the frontal projection has been often described as egg shaped. This configuration, which occurs, however, in only about 50% of the cases, is due to the combined effects of a narrow base, increased prominence of the right heart border from right atrial enlargement, and prominence of the left heart border as well as inferior-leftward displacement of the cardiac apex from left ventricular enlargement.

Since the anteriorly situated right ventricle harbors systemic pressures, right ventricular hypertrophy is almost always observed in the electrocardiogram and vectorcardiogram. During the 1st week of life, however, the tracings may appear normal although inversion of the T waves in the left precordial leads is not uncommon. In CTGA with IVS, left ventricular hypertrophy is generally not observed since the posteriorly situated left ventricle has relatively low pressures. On the other hand, combined ven-

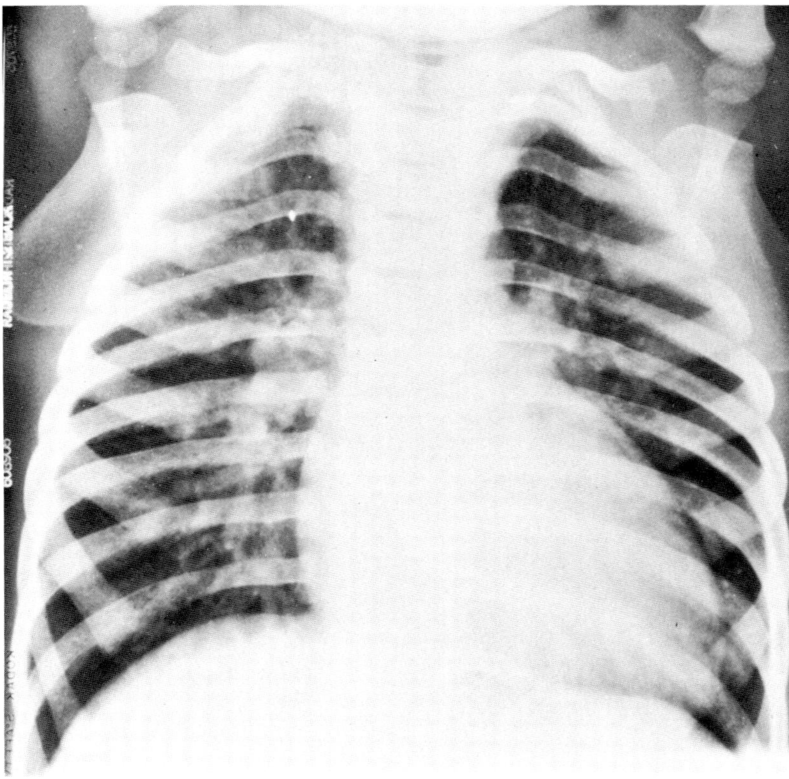

Figure 6. Chest roentgenogram in frontal projection of a 21-month-old infant with CTGA and IVS who had successful Rashkind atrioseptotomy palliation at age 14 days.

tricular hypertrophy is not unusual in CTGA with VSD. In the presence of associated pulmonary stenosis, there may also be left ventricular hypertrophy in about 25% of the cases in addition to the right ventricular hypertrophy. Right atrial enlargement may be observed later in infancy. Left atrial enlargement may also be noted in those with VSD and minimal atrial shunting, i.e., in those with clearly left atrial volume overload.

The diagnosis is established by cardiac catheterization and angiocardiography. The various objectives in the performance of this diagnostic procedure are summarized in Figure 4. The abnormal origin of the great vessels is suspected from the unusual catheter positions as shown, but the diagnosis is confirmed by angiocardiography which shows the anterior aorta arising from the right ventricle, and the posterior pulmonary trunk from the left ventricle (Fig. 7, A and B). An atrial septal defect is demonstrated by shunting of contrast media from left atrium to right atrium

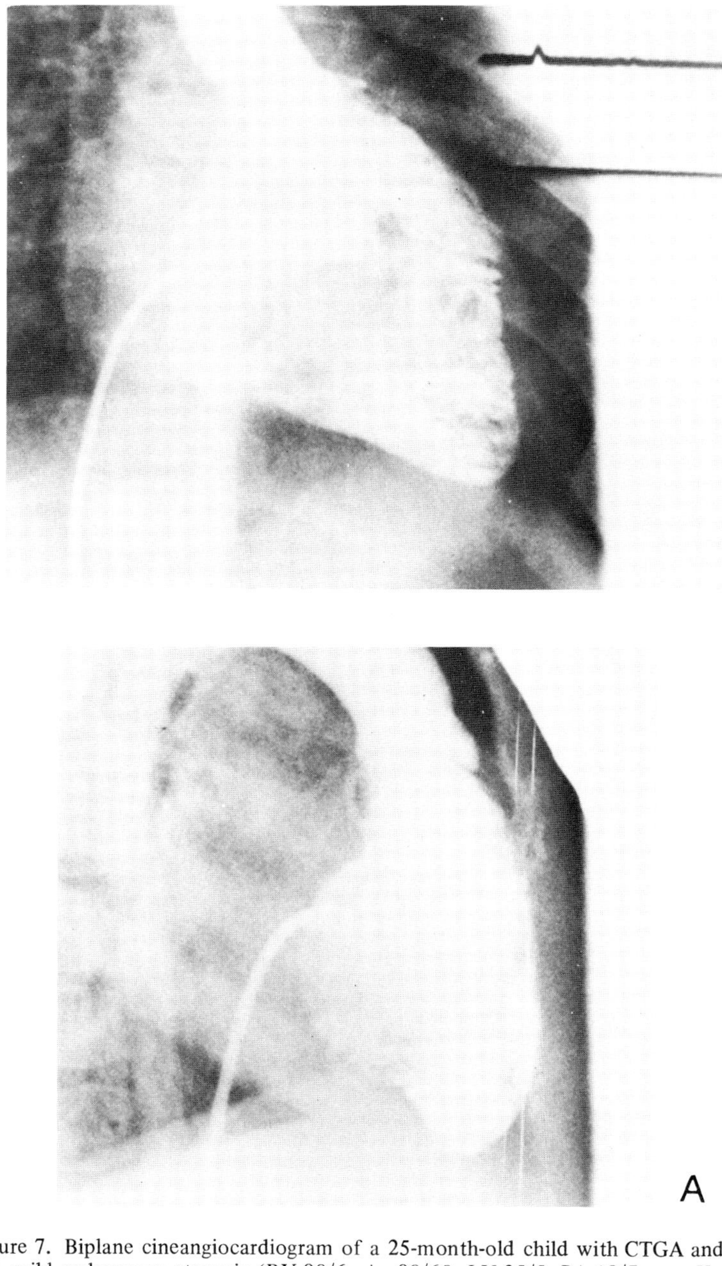

A

Figure 7. Biplane cineangiocardiogram of a 25-month-old child with CTGA and IVS and mild pulmonary stenosis (RV-90/6, Ao-90/60, LV-35/5, PA-18/7 mm. Hg). A. Frontal and lateral projection cineframes following contrast injection into right ventricle. B. Frontal and lateral projection cineframes following contrast injection into left ventricle. Note mild narrowing at subvalvar region in the lateral projection.

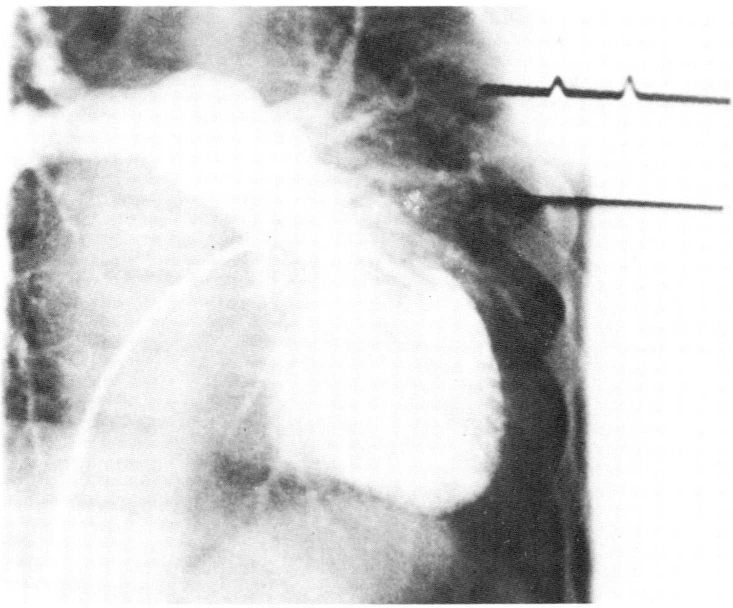

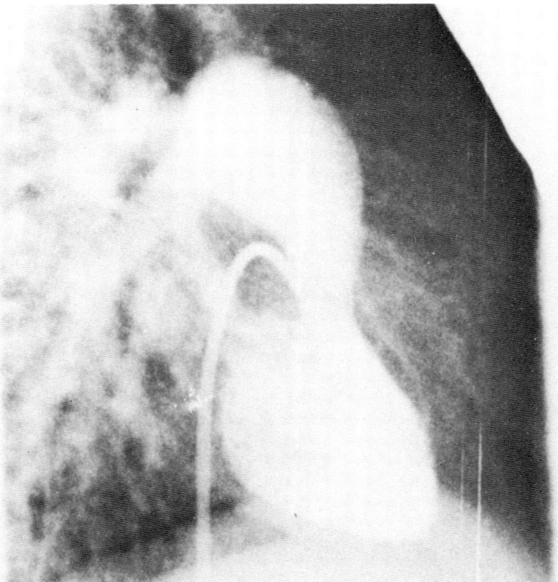

B

following injection into the pulmonary artery or left ventricle. Left ventricular outflow obstruction (pulmonary stenosis) is also shown by the left ventricular angiocardiograms, as well as by the continuous pressure recording from pulmonary artery to left ventricle demonstrating a significant systolic pressure gradient. A ventricular septal defect is readily demonstrated by shunting of contrast material from right ventricle to left ventricle after its injection into the right ventricle. The origins of the coronary arteries are abnormal (9, 10). The right coronary artery generally arises from the posterior aortic sinus, while the left coronary artery originates from the left anterior sinus. The non-coronary sinus is thus situated anteriorly and to the right. Occasionally, the left circumflex artery is a branch of the right coronary artery or arises separately also from the posterior sinus. Bronchial blood flow is difficult to assess quantitatively but it sometimes appears prominent especially in those with pulmonary stenosis (Fig. 8).

In addition to establishing the primary diagnosis, including the cardiac shunting or mixing sites, cardiac catheterization is also designed to evaluate the size and function of both ventricles, and especially the status of the pulmonary circulation in terms of its pressure, flow, and vascular resistance. Pulmonary blood flow calculation in CTGA is not as reliable as in other forms of heart diseases due to failure to estimate the contribution of bronchial flow upon the total pulmonary flow (11), the unsteady basal and metabolic state of the sick infant, and difficulties in estimating oxygen consumption in such small subjects. It is also not always possible to enter the pulmonary artery. In this case, blood samples obtained from the left ventricle do not reliably reflect those of the pulmonary arteries due to inadequate or poor mixing of blood in the ventricle. Nevertheless, pulmonary and systemic flows have been estimated using the standard Fick method, and these have been shown to be increased in both circuits (5). As discussed earlier, the calculated effective pulmonary blood flow reflects the degree of intercirculatory mixing. This has been estimated to be often limited in CTGA (12, 13). It is considered inadequate when the EPBF is less than 1.0 L/min./$M^2$, and especially when less than 0.7 L/min./$M^2$. Following successful palliation by balloon septotomy or atrial septectomy, or in the presence of a good sized atrial septal defect or VSD, the EPBF is often on the order of 1.5 to 2.0 L/min./$M^2$ or even higher.

Because of the peculiar arrangement of the two circuits, in parallel rather than in series, the usual practice of expressing the relative magnitudes of the pulmonary blood flow (Qp) and systemic blood flow (Qs) in the form of a Qp/Qs ratio is not valid. By the same token, it is not too useful or, in fact, may be misleading, to express pulmonary vascular resistance (Rp) relative to systemic vascular resistance (Rs) in the form of

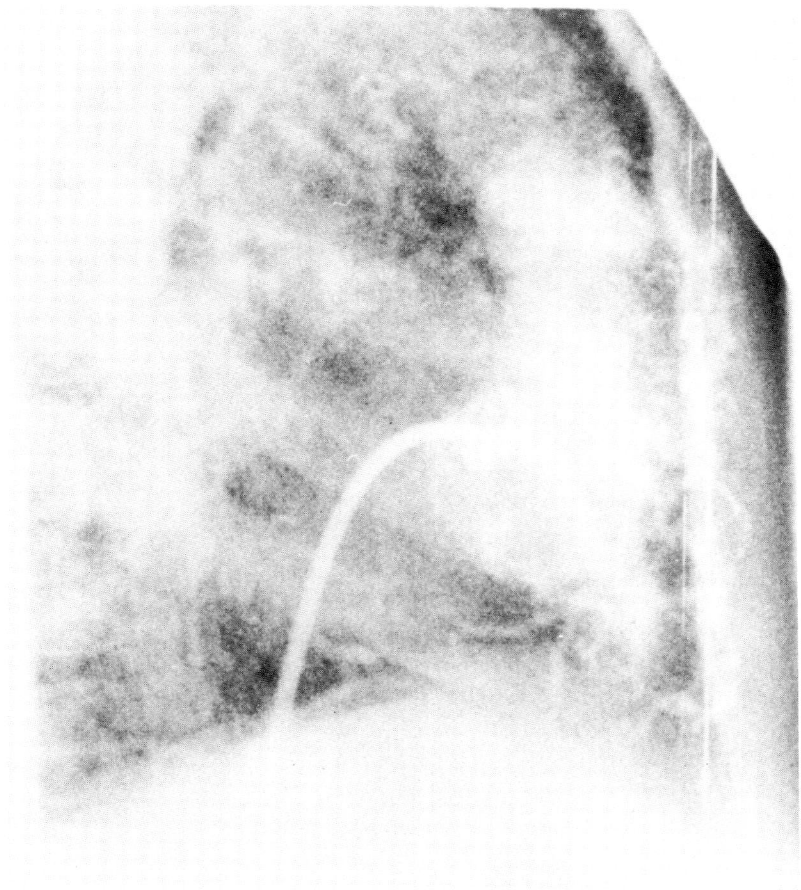

Figure 8. Cineframe of same angiocardiogram in Figure 7, demonstrating abundant bronchial vessels. Increased bronchial circulation was confirmed at time of open-heart surgery.

a Rp/Rs ratio (12). The severity of the pulmonary arteriolar resistance is expressed more meaningfully by the absolute value that is calculated: Rp of over 10.0 units/$M^2$ (800 dynes sec. $cm.^{-5}/M^2$) is, generally speaking, already accompanied by significant pulmonary vascular changes and obstruction (7, 12).

The pulmonary artery pressure in CTGA with IVS is usually only mildly or moderately elevated or sometimes within the normal range, and the pulmonary (or left ventricular)/aortic systolic pressure ratio is often in the range of 0.30 to 0.50. This relatively low pulmonary pressure state does not appear to change with age. In exceptional instances, however, marked pulmonary hypertension may be observed, for reasons not clear. In contrast, the pulmonary artery pressures are generally in the systemic range when CTGA is accompanied by a significantly large VSD (10, 13, 14). If pulmonary stenosis is present, the pulmonary artery pressure may be normal or elevated depending on the severity of the left ventricular outflow obstruction. Also, if the VSD is small or is absent, the left ventricular pressure may only be mildly elevated provided that the pulmonary stenosis is mild.

Paul and associates (14) have demonstrated that pulmonary vascular resistance remains within normal limits over an age range extending from infancy through 10 years in CTGA with IVS, or in those with pulmonary stenosis. On the other hand, increased pulmonary resistance is observed in CTGA with significant-sized VSD as early as the 1st year, and this appears to progress fairly rapidly in subsequent years. These observations are shown schematically in Figure 9, which also illustrates the corresponding progression of the pulmonary vascular disease with age.

Right and left ventricular function can also be evaluated by determining the ventricular volumes angiocardiographically during end-diastole and during end-systole. Other derived parameters such as stroke volume, ejection fraction, and left ventricular mass can also be derived (15, 16). Of special interest is the long-term performance evaluation of the right ventricle from infancy through childhood after successful surgery, to determine how well and for how long it can remain an effective systemic ventricle. Such an investigation includes the determination of myocardial "contractility" through analysis of the isovolumic phase of ventricular contraction as derived from high fidelity pressure recordings using catheter-tip microtransducers (17) (Fig. 10).

## MANAGEMENT

Depending largely on the associated defects, severe cardiac failure may occur during the 1st or 2nd week of life, by the 2nd month, or after infancy (Fig. 11). The circulatory failure in the early newborn period is usually secondary to gross inadequacy of the intercirculatory mixing such as in CTGA with IVS, where shunting occurs chiefly across a patent foramen ovale or small atrial septal defect plus a small or closing ductus arteriosus. In the babies in whom the heart failure is somewhat delayed and of comparatively slower onset, progressing in severity till it peaks sometime during or after the 2nd month, a large VSD is usually present, resulting in excessive pulmonary flow and marked pulmonary hypertension. In the non-surgically treated subjects, survival after the 1st year

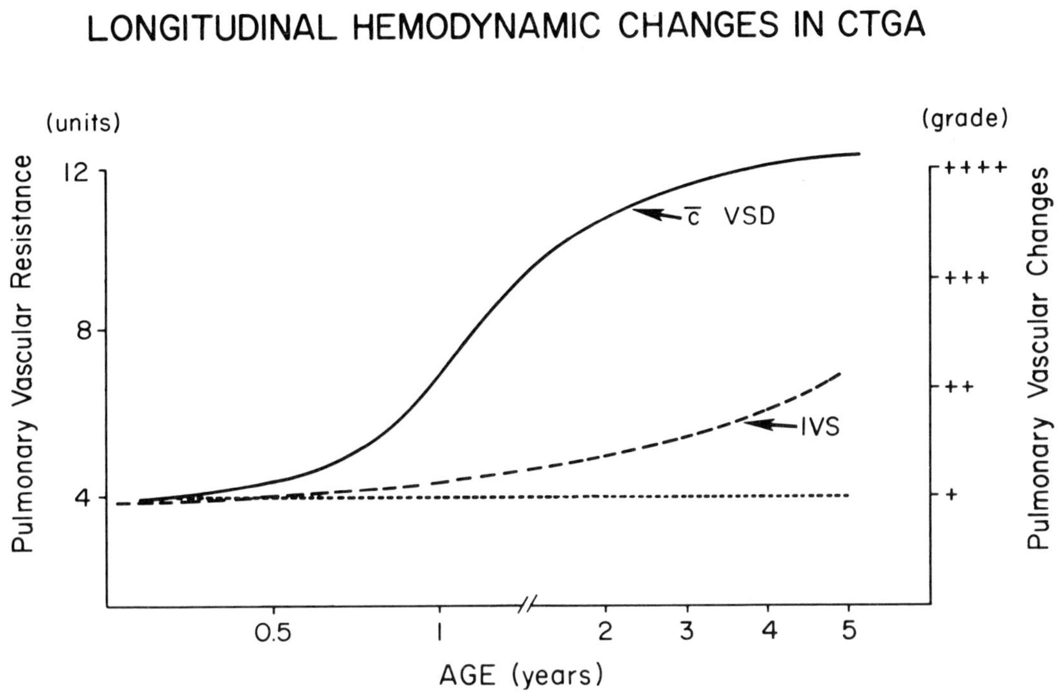


Figure 9. Time course of pulmonary vascular resistance and of pulmonary vascular disease, shown schematically, in infants and children with CTGA and IVS, and in those with CTGA and VSD.

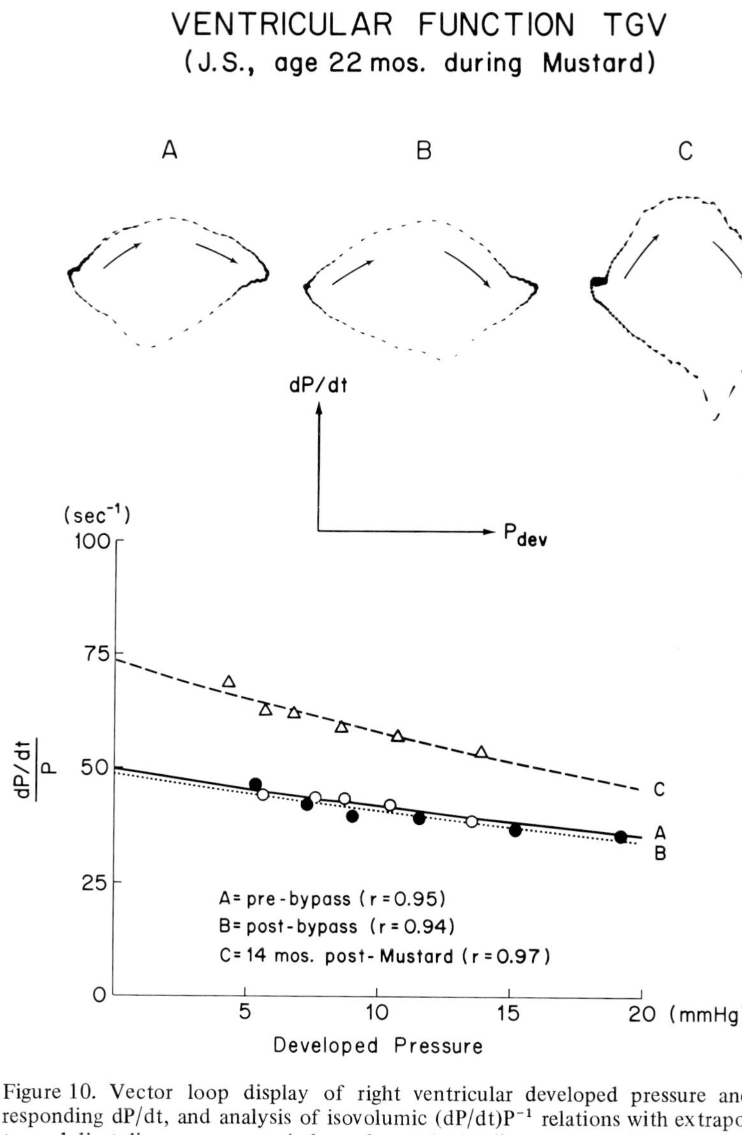


Figure 10. Vector loop display of right ventricular developed pressure and corresponding dP/dt, and analysis of isovolumic $(dP/dt)P^{-1}$ relations with extrapolation to end-diastolic pressure, as index of ventricular "contractility." First two dP/dt loops were obtained at time of surgery, before and after the Mustard operation; third loop was taken during cardiac catheterization several months later.

occurs in only about 10 to 20% (4, 10). These are generally those with IVS and large atrial septal defect, or those with VSD and mild to moderate pulmonary stenosis. In these as well as in the surgically palliated subjects,

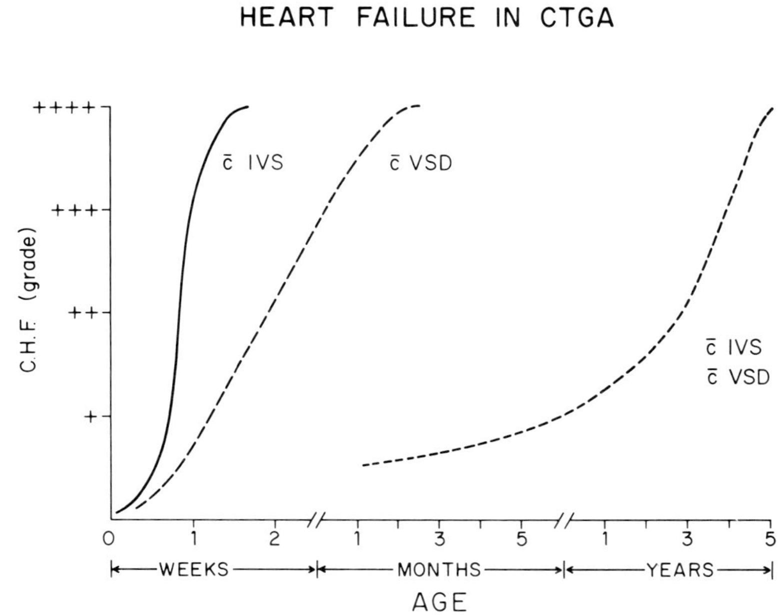


Figure 11. Usual time events for heart failure and death in surgically untreated CTGA illustrated schematically.

death from the complications from long standing polycythemia, heart failure, pulmonary disease, brain abscess, or bacterial endocarditis may occur several years later.

It is obvious from the foregoing discussion that early diagnosis is critical in the management of CTGA. Even before cardiac catheterization, correction of the acidotic state with sodium bicarbonate, although resulting in temporary relief only, is essential. If blood gas data are available, 0.5 mEq/kg. body weight may be given intravenously for each mEq/L of base deficit. In a desperately ill baby, poorly responsive and with ashen grey color, acidosis can be assumed to be present, and sodium bicarbonate may be given empirically using an initial dose of 2 to 3 mEq/kg. The subsequent doses will depend on the blood gas findings. Maintenance of a normal body temperature is also essential. The usual medical measures consisting of oxygen, digitalis, and, sometimes, diuretics are instituted whenever cardiac failure is suspected. At the time of cardiac catheterization, and immediately after the demonstration of CTGA, atrial septotomy (Rashkind procedure) is carried out using a balloon catheter advanced into the left atrium. Once identified to be inside this chamber, the balloon is inflated with 2.0 to 2.5 ml. contrast medium-saline mixture, and then rapidly withdrawn in a sharp, jerky motion into the right atrium-inferior caval junction. This is repeated several times until any resistance to balloon traversal across the atrial septum has disappeared. The inflated balloon usually has a diameter of nearly 1.5 cm., and the resulting septal tear often has a diameter of approximately 1.0 cm.

Balloon septotomy results not only in increased intercirculatory mixing but also in left atrial and pulmonary venous decompression as left to right atrial shunting is enhanced. The former effect is reflected by an immediate rise in systemic arterial oxygen saturation. The latter is shown by disappearance or significant reduction of any pre-existing interatrial pressure gradient following a drop in left atrial pressure. In addition, there is an immediate and dramatic change in respiration consisting of disappearance of the tachypnea that has been present all along. The change in respiration is accompanied by an improvement in pulmonary compliance as pulmonary venous congestion is relieved (Fig. 12).

It should be pointed out that absence of a significant pressure gradient between the two atria, noted initially at the time of cardiac catheterization, does not necessarily assure presence of a functionally large interatrial communication since venous return to both atria, whose distensibility are intrinsically different, may vary. Thus left atrial pressure may not be much higher than that of the right atrium if pulmonary venous return into the former is comparatively much less than that returning into the right atrium. In other words, atrial septotomy should be attempted in practically every subject with CTGA especially in the newborn period. Our experience is similar to those of others (14, 18, 19) who have shown successful immediate and long-term (over 8 to 12 months) palliation by the Rashkind procedure in about 80 to 90%. Whereas this high degree of success is observed when the procedure is done on newborn subjects, the likelihood of good palliation drops when carried out on infants over 1 or 2 months of age. In those where effective palliation has not been achieved, or where atrial crossflow appears to have decreased over a period of weeks or months after the initial improvement, surgical creation of an atrial septal defect (Blalock-Hanlon procedure) is done for the same purpose. The rise in systemic arterial oxygen saturation following this surgical procedure is greater than that which follows the Rashkind procedure.

The management of CTGA with VSD differs somewhat from that of CTGA with IVS since the threat of a rapidly progressing pulmonary vascular obstructive disease is real in the former (Fig. 9). Although atrial septotomy or septectomy is helpful for left atrial decompression, heart failure generally persists and requires intensive medical therapy. Not infrequently, palliative surgical banding of the pulmonary artery is done at age few months not only to control the heart failure but also to reduce

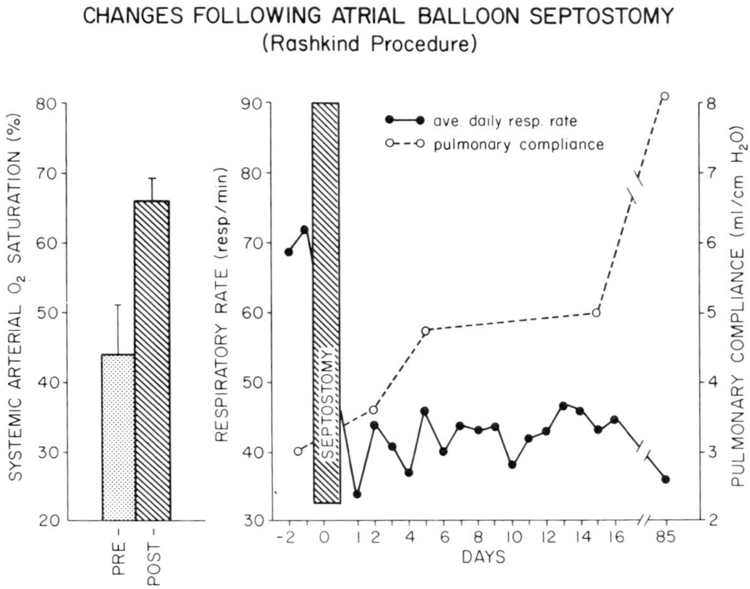


Figure 12. Changes in systemic arterial oxygen saturation, respiratory rate and pulmonary compliance following Rashkind procedure. The bar graphs at left demonstrate the mean ± S.D. of aortic $O_2$ saturation in 14 newborn infants before and immediately after atrioseptotomy. The graph on the right, taken from a baby with CTGA and IVS, shows the typical changes in respiration and in pulmonary compliance following successful palliation.

pulmonary hypertension and the likelihood of future pulmonary vascular obstruction. "Corrective" surgery, using the Mustard procedure, can then be performed after infancy. Whether the pulmonary artery banding should also be done, for reasons already given, on those where the heart failure has responded favorably to medical therapy, or whether the Mustard operation should instead be carried out at an earlier age than usual, such as some time in the latter half of infancy, is still an unresolved question. Although admittedly meager, there is some surgical risk involved in pulmonary artery banding. In addition, there are some potential undesirable sequelae such as acquired left ventricular outflow obstruction persisting even after debanding or restricted growth of the pulmonary annulus with consequent stenosis. On the other hand, the Mustard procedure done at age 2 or more years is technically easier and offers a greater chance of long-term success than that done during infancy. Pulmonary artery banding is generally not necessary in CTGA with IVS.

The cerebrovascular accidents which sometimes occur in CTGA and other forms of cyanotic congenital heart disease are often due to venous or arterial thromboses and cerebral infarctions. Occasionally, there may be hemorrhagic diathesis due to a variety of coagulation abnormalities such as thrombocytopenia, hypofibrinogenemia, prolonged prothrombin or thromboplastin generation time, or deficiency of some of the plasma clotting factors (21), which may enhance the likelihood of cerebral hemorrhage in the presence of these thromboembolic changes.

The incidence of these neurologic complications in CTGA have varied from 2.4 to a high 17.7% (10, 18, 21). With increased utilization of palliative procedures, its occurrence rate appears to have dropped. Analysis of the hematologic picture of children who have developed these complications has shown that the children below 4 years of age revealed not only hypoxemia and some polycythemia but also low mean corpuscular hemoglobin concentration, indicating relative anemia. By contrast, the neurologic complications in the older children occurred in the presence of marked polycythemia and normal or elevated mean corpuscular hemoglobin concentration (21, 22). These findings suggest that cerebrovascular accidents in cyanotic congenital heart disease may be minimized if the candidates for these complications are properly identified and appropriately treated. Young subjects with relative anemia should be on oral iron therapy unless the hematocrit has reached dangerously high levels of 60 to 65% or greater. In the older subjects with marked polycythemia and hematocrit of nearly 65% or more, erythroperesis consisting of incremental volume for volume exchange of whole blood with plasmanate or with 5% human albumin in physiologic saline solution is done until an ideal venous hematocrit of approximately 55% is achieved. In the absence of pulmonary stenosis, the procedure results in an immediate increase in systemic and pulmonary flow, and in corresponding drop in systemic as well as pulmonary vascular resistances (24). How long these hemodynamic effects remain is not known. Peripheral blood flow studies, using venous occlusion plethysmography, have shown that the initial significant improvement in peripheral flow is followed by gradual return to the pre-erythropheresis levels over a period of usually 4 to 8 weeks (24). Erythropheresis is, therefore, useful only for transient relief.

A better therapeutic approach for the correction of the high polycythemia and its potential complications should be directed at primarily correcting the hypoxemic state by surgery, either palliative atrial septectomy or the Mustard procedure. In CTGA with VSD and significant pulmonary stenosis, the plasmanate/blood exchange results in increased systemic flow but reduced pulmonary flow and corresponding drop in systemic arterial oxygen saturation (23).

There has been considerable progress in the management of CTGA. The introduction of the Rashkind procedure (or the Blalock-Hanlon procedure) for creating an interatrial communication as early as in the immediate newborn period has unquestionably accounted for a high salvage rate of newborn infants who would have naturally died at this early age. The Mustard procedure, aimed at correcting the transposed arterial anomaly by creating a corresponding transposed venous return to the heart, has been most gratifying. However, by this approach, the right ventricle is allowed to continue to function as the systemic ventricle while the left ventricle serves as the pulmonary ventricle. The fate of the right ventricle in this unusual role must await the test of time. There are some disturbing observations which suggest that right ventricular performance is not quite normal under this setting. The future of the intra-atrial baffle used to realign venous return to the opposite ventricles also remains to be seen. It should be emphasized that these successfully corrected children remain potential candidates for infective bacterial endocarditis. They should, therefore, be submitted to the usual antibiotic prophylactic regime whenever subjected to dental work or other surgical procedures.

## REFERENCES


1. Lambert, E. C., Canent, R. V., and Hohn, A. R. 1966. Congenital cardiac anomalies in the newborn: a review of conditions causing death or severe distress in the first month of life. Pediatrics 37: 343–351.
2. Rowe, R. D. and Mehrizi, A. 1968. The Neonate With Congenital Heart Disease, p. 80. Saunders, Philadelphia.
3. Carlgren, L. 1959. The incidence of congenital heart disease in children born in Gothenburg 1941–1950. Br. Heart J. 21: 40–50.
4. Liebman, J., Cullun, L., and Belloc, N. B. 1969. Natural history of transposition of the great arteries: anatomy and birth and death characteristics. Circulation 40: 237–262.
5. Mair, D. D. and Ritter, D. G. 1972. Factors influencing intercirculatory mixing in patients with complete transposition of the great arteries. Am. J. Cardiol. 30: 653–658.
6. Viles, Ph. H., Ongley, P. A., and Titus, J. L. 1969. The spectrum of pulmonary vascular disease in transposition of the great arteries. Circulation 40: 31–41.
7. Newfield, E. A., Muster, A. J., Paul, M., and Idriss, F. S. 1974. Pulmonary vascular disease in complete transposition of the great arteries: A study of 200 patients. Am. J. Cardiol. 34: 75–82.
8. Replogle, R. L., Mieselman, H. J., and Merrill, E. W. 1967. Clinical implications of blood rheology studies. Circulation 36: 148–160.
9. Rowlatt, U. F. 1962. Coronary artery distribution in complete transpostion. J. Am. Med. Assoc. 179: 269–278.
10. Shaher, R. M. 1973. Complete Transposition Of The Great Arteries. Academic Press, New York.

11. Burchell, H. B. 1966. Some hemodynamic problems in transposition of the great vessels (edit). Circulation 33: 181–182.
12. Mair, D. D., Ritter, D. G., Ongley, P. A., and Helmholz, H. F., Jr. 1971. Hemodynamics and evaluation for surgery of patients with complete transposition of the great arteries and ventricular septal defect. Am. J. Cardiol. 28: 632–640.
13. Shaher, R. M. 1964. The hemodynamics of complete transposition of the great vessels. Br. Heart J. 26: 343–353.
14. Paul, M. H. 1971. Transposition of the great arteries: physiologic data. *In* The Natural History And Progress In Treatment Of Congenital Heart Defects. Kidd, B. S. L. and Keith, J. D. (Eds.), p. 144. Charles C. Thomas, Springfield, Illinois.
15. Graham T. P., Jarmakani, J. M., Canent, R. V., Jr., and Jewett, P. H. 1971. Quantitation of left heart volume and systolic output in transposition of the great arteries. Circulation 44: 899–909.
16. Thilenius, O. G. and Arcilla, R. A. 1973. Ventricular volume in transposition of the great vessels with intact ventricular septum (TGV). Pediat. Res. 7: 299.
17. Arcilla, R. A., Sodt, P., and Replogle, R. 1974. Vector display of cardiac performance: A new approach for evaluating ventricular function. Cardiology 59: 102–113.
18. Rashkind, W. J. 1971. Transposition of the great arteries. Pediatr. Clin. North Am. 18: 1075–1090.
19. Rashkind, W. J. and Miller, W. W. 1968. Transposition of the great arteries; results of palliation by balloon atrioseptostomy in 31 infants. Circulation 38: 453–462.
20. Ekert, H., Gilchrist, G. S., and Stanton, R. 1970. Hemostasis in cyanotic congenital heart disease. J. Pediatr. 76: 221–230.
21. Phornphutkul, C., Rosenthal, A., Nadas, A. S., and Berenberg, W. 1973. Cerebrovascular accidents in infants and children with cyanotic congenital heart disease. Am. J. Cardiol. 32: 329–334.
22. Tyler, H. R. and Clark, D. B. 1957. Cerebrovascular accidents in patients with congenital heart disease. Arch. Neurol. Psychiatr. 77: 483–489.
23. Rosenthal, A. and Fyler, D. C. 1974. Effect of red cell volume reduction on pulmonary blood flow in polycythemia of cyanotic congenital heart disease. Am. J. Cardiol. 33: 410–414.
24. Cassels, D. Personal communication.

# 7 Surgical Treatment of Transposition of the Great Arteries: Technical Considerations and Results

D. A. Cooley, M.D.

While surgeons had been challenged earlier to find a method for surgical treatment of transposition of the great arteries (TGA), the report by Hanlon and Blalock (1) in 1948 first provided a useful technique for palliative treatment. Their technique of atrial septectomy was first used in our hospital in 1954 and was subsequently modified to reduce the operative complications, notably pulmonary consolidation and hemorrhagic edema (Fig. 1). We also emphasized the need for early operation in newborn infants since death within the first few weeks is common (2, 3). It is well known that those infants without a naturally occurring shunt (atrial septal defect, ventricular septal defect or patent ductus arteriosus) are most susceptible to early death. Therefore palliative treatment must be done in those patients during the first few days or weeks of life.

Since that early beginning of surgical treatment for transposition two major developments have appeared: one for nonoperative palliation and the other for a surgical "cure." In 1966 Rashkind and Miller (4) introduced the technique of balloon septostomy in which the cardiologist performing the initial diagnostic cardiac catheterization may provide a therapeutic addition to the study. Forceful withdrawal of an inflated

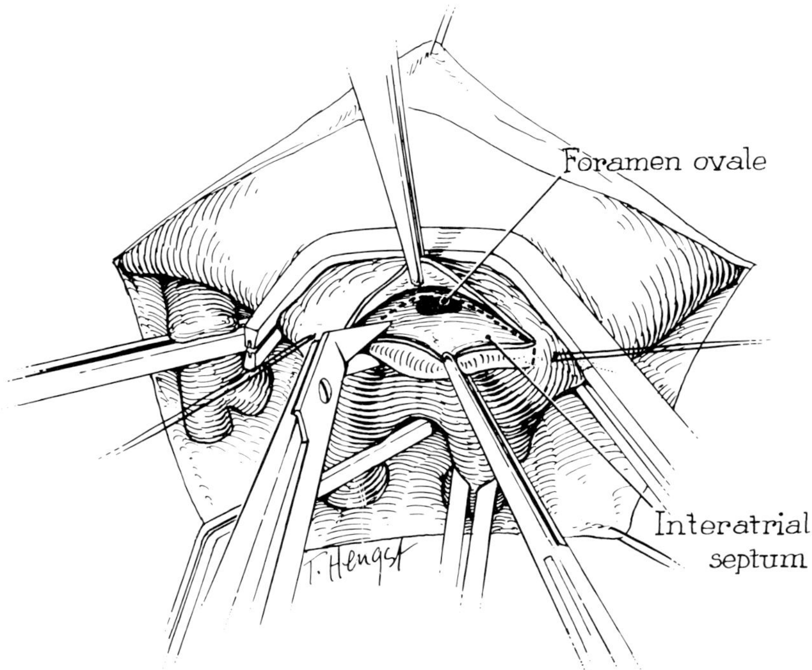


Figure 1. Drawing showing modified technique of Blalock-Hanlon atrial septectomy removing a large segment of septum. The right pulmonary veins are attached on the right atrial wall enhancing the repair later with a Mustard procedure. Pulmonary veins are temporarily clamped and the right pulmonary artery should also be occluded to prevent pulmonary congestion during the period of venous occlusion.

balloon tip catheter from the left atrium to the right atrium ruptures the membranous partition of the fossa ovalis. Immediate improvement occurs in saturation of arterial blood, usually a 10 to 20% increase.

Ten years after Albert (5) described a technique of direct repair, Mustard (6) applied a similar technique successfully in patients. Complications of this ingenious operation were encountered, consisting mainly of conduction disturbances and obstruction to venous inflow into the revised atria. The high incidence of conduction disturbances was related to injury of the sinoatrial node and interruption of intra-atrial conduction pathways (Fig. 2) (7). Both have been almost eliminated by modifications of the original technique described by Mustard. In the original method the coronary sinus was opened widely and the coronary venous blood was directed into the new "right" atrium beneath the atrial baffle. At present the accepted technique is to leave the coronary sinus intact and permit the unoxygenated blood to enter the chamber receiving pulmonary venous

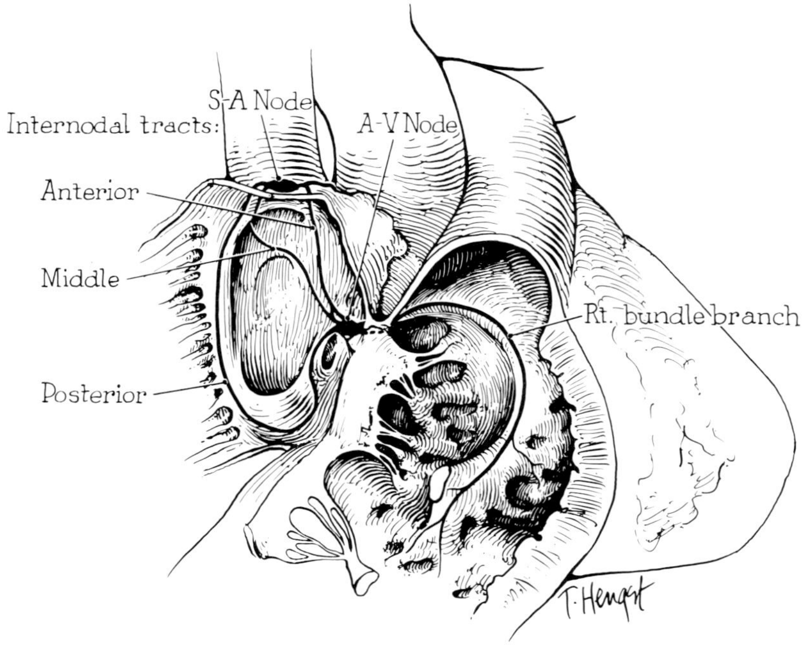


Figure 2. Drawing showing the location of internodal conduction pathways between the sinoatrial and atrioventricular nodes. An incision uncovering the coronary sinus could interrupt all three causing various abnormal cardiac arrhythmias.

blood. The reduction in systemic saturation is slight and is a small disadvantage compared to the dysrhythmia associated with the original technique. Insertion of the superior caval cannula directly into the superior vena cava rather than through an atrial pursestring suture avoids injury in this crucial area and gives the surgeon an unobstructed view of the atrial cavities.

Postoperative obstruction to venous return, either pulmonary or systemic, may be prevented in several ways. The baffle should be made from autologous pericardium since Dacron has proved unsatisfactory in our experience (8, 9). The baffle, rather than being rectangular as originally described, should be dumbbell shaped or, as described by Brom (10), shaped like a pair of pantaloons or trousers (Fig. 3). The experienced surgeon can avoid technical errors which may cause obstruction of the vena cavae or pulmonary veins. When the passage from the pulmonary to the new "left" atrium is unusually narrow as is common in infants or patients who have never undergone septectomy, a "gore" or patch of woven Dacron or pericardium should be inserted into the stenosed area

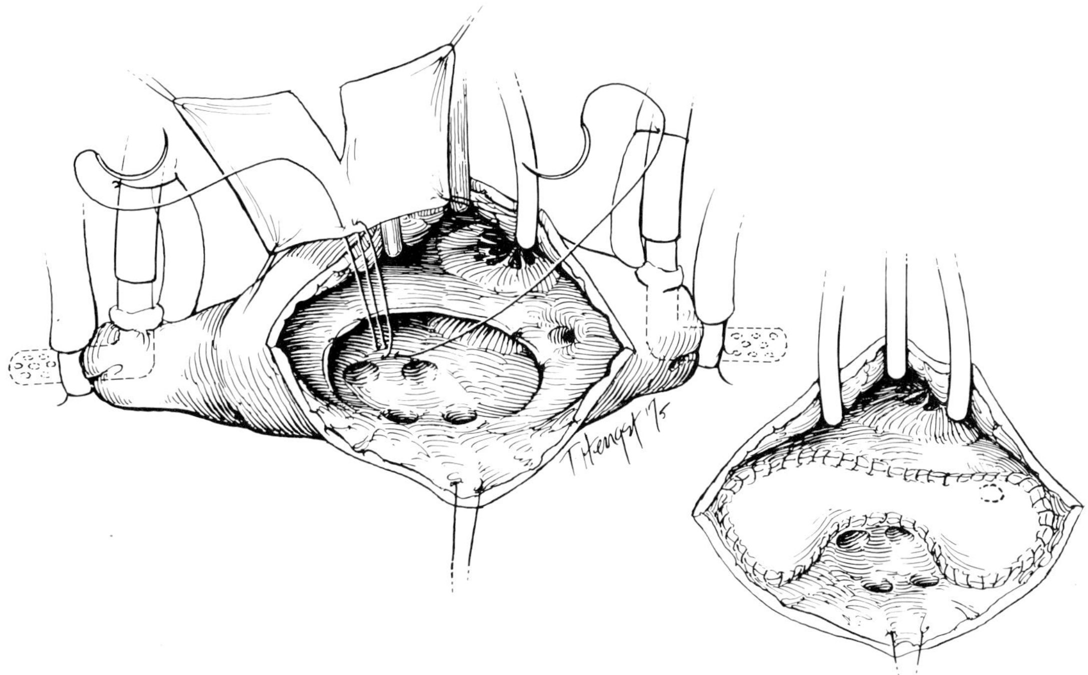

Figure 3. Drawing showing technique of modified Mustard repair. The superior vena caval catheter is introduced directly into the cava avoiding injury to the sinoatrial node. The pericardial baffle has a "pantaloon" shape. The coronary sinus is intact with coronary venous blood directed into the new systemic atrial and ventricular cavities.

after making an incision between the superior and inferior orifices. The incision may be extended through the crista terminalis without causing conduction disturbances or other complications (8).

A large ventricular septal defect (VSD) in a patient with TGA frequently leads to severe pulmonary hypertension during childhood, and the pulmonary vascular resistance usually increases with age. Complete correction in such patients may carry a high or prohibitive risk. In such cases palliative treatment without attempting closure of the VSD may provide a good alternative. Recently in selected patients of older age with a large VSD and elevated pulmonary arterial pressure without extremely high pulmonary vascular resistance, we have performed a Mustard operation without closure of the VSD. Systemic arterial oxygen saturation should increase strikingly and excellent palliation is achieved. The concept of the palliative Mustard operation is to convert a severely cyanotic patient with TGA and VSD to a mildly cyanotic patient with only VSD, akin to the Eisenmenger complex. The quality of life is substantially improved and prognosis and life expectancy are increased.

Considered anatomically inoperable were those patients with TGA, a large VSD, and in some instances pulmonary stenosis. If the VSD was closed even with a patch graft, the outlet from the left ventricle was obstructed. Rastelli and co-workers (11) recommended a technique in which the VSD is covered with a patch graft as a tunnel which diverts blood from the left ventricle to the aorta. The pulmonary valve is then closed and a composite tube graft containing a heterograft or homograft valve is used to provide continuity between the right ventricle and pulmonary artery (Fig. 4). This technique may be useful in such complex situations. In rare instances normal pulmonary and aortic valves override the interventricular septum with the pulmonary valve facing more to the left and the aortic to the right. Under these conditions a baffle or tunnel of pericardium placed in spiral fashion may redirect left ventricular blood to the aorta and right ventricular blood to the pulmonary artery (12). Methods are being studied to correct simple TGA by a direct means by transferring the pulmonary and aortic valves. Moving the coronary ostia with the aortic root remains a problem which may be solved by applying newer techniques of microvascular surgery (13, 14, 15).

## RESULTS

Experience with TGA at the Texas Children's Hospital and the Texas Heart Institute embraces a 20-year period beginning in 1954 and includes approximately 450 surgical procedures. Techniques of medical and surgical

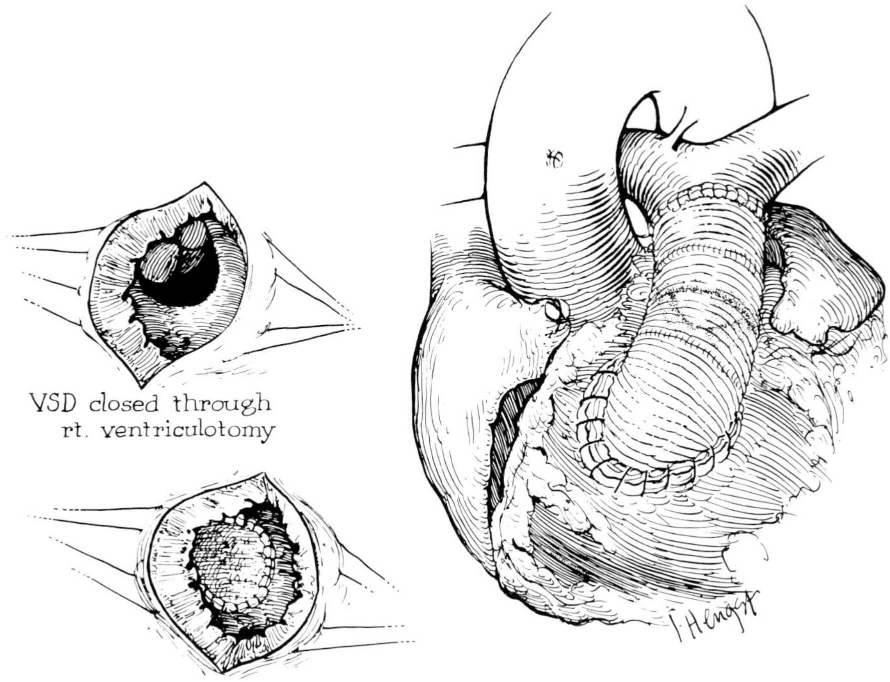


Figure 4. Drawing showing a method of repair of TGA with a large VSD and pulmonary valvular or subvalvular obstruction. The VSD is repaired with a large patch of knitted Dacron placing the aorta in continuity with the left ventricle. Right ventricle-to-pulmonary arterial continuity is obtained with a composite Dacron graft containing a hetero- or homograft semilunar valve.

management have changed almost continuously during that period. At present three treatment methods are in general use and results will be presented separately although overlap of data is unavoidable.

## Balloon Septostomy (Rashkind)

Results were recently reported from Texas Children's Hospital by Gutgessel and McNamara (16) and included all patients with dextro TGA who underwent balloon atrial septostomy (BAS) between September 1967 and December 1972. BAS was used in all infants at the initial cardiac catheterization. Age at time of BAS ranged from 1 day to 5 months; 80% of the infants were under 1 month of age. Of 62 patients, 34 (55%) had simple TGA, 13 (21%) had a large VSD, 13 (21%) had pulmonary stenosis (PS), and 2 (3%) had both VSD and PS. Six of 62 patients also had patent ductus arteriosus and one had coarctation of the aorta. The report included an evaluation of patients through December 1973 providing a 1- to 6-year longitudinal study.

PS was considered to be present if there was a peak systolic pressure gradient in excess of 35 mm. Hg or if there was angiographic evidence of left ventricular outflow obstruction. VSD was considered to be large if equal pressures were found between the two ventricles in the absence of PS. Two patients with a small VSD were included with simple TGA.

Early results of BAS were classified as follows:

1. *Good result:* An increase in saturation of systemic arterial blood greater than 10 percentage points, a residual mean interatrial pressure gradient of less than 2 mm. Hg, and definite clinical improvement.
2. *Fair result:* An increase in oxygen saturation less than 10%, a persistent atrial pressure gradient of 2 to 4 mm. Hg, and only slight clinical improvement.
3. *Unsatisfactory result:* No increase in systemic oxygen saturation, a residual atrial mean pressure gradient of more than 4 mm. Hg, lack of clinical improvement, or BAS-related death.

Late results of BAS were classified as "good" when survival to 6 months of age with an arterial saturation greater than 60% was recorded; anything less was "unsatisfactory." Many patients with VSD and TGA frequently have a saturation of 60% or more without BAS; only the patients without VSD (intact septum) were classified in this way.

By the end of the study, survivors had been followed for an average of 37 months after BAS (range, 12 to 72 months). Fifty-five (89%) of the 62 patients had either a "good" or a fair early result (Table I). The four unsatisfactory results included four deaths: one instance of perforation of the right atrium and fatal pericardial tamponade, one of fatal arrhythmia produced by BAS, one death from congestive heart failure and one death during induction of anesthesia for emergency ligation of a patent ductus arteriosus and pulmonary banding following BAS. Three other deaths were unclassified. Of 43 patients analyzed as late results, 25 (58%) had good results (i.e., lived 6 months, had no stroke, and an oxygen saturation over 60%).

Thirty-two patients in this series underwent subsequent palliative operations. Twenty had Blalock-Hanlon atrial septectomy either alone or with other palliative procedures and one death occurred. The mortality of all palliative operations was 9% (3 of 32 operations) with all deaths occurring in patients under two months of age. Thirty-one patients underwent Mustard repair during the time of the study and eight (26%) died (Table II). No deaths occurred in patients more than 24 months old.

Table I. Results of Balloon Atrial Septostomy (from Gutgesell & McNamara (16))

| | Total No. of Patients | TGA[a] (Simple) | PS[a] | VSD[a] | PS + VSD |
|---|---|---|---|---|---|
| Early results | | | | | |
| Good | 47 (76%) | 25 | 13 | 7 | 2 |
| Fair | 8 (13%) | 5 | | 3 | |
| Unsatisfactory (died) | 4 ( 6%) | 1 | | 3 | |
| Not classified | 3 ( 5%) | 3 | | | |
| | 62 | 34 | 13 | 13 | 2 |
| Late results[b] | | | | | |
| Good | 25 (58%) | 16 | 9 | | |
| Unsatisfactory | 18 (42%) | 14 | 4 | | |
| | 43 | 30 | 13 | | |

[a]TGA = transposition of the great arteries; PS = pulmonic stenosis; VSD = ventricular septal defect.

[b]Includes only patients with an early "good" or "fair" balloon atrial septostomy result. Patients with VSD or VSD and PS were not included because the criteria were not applicable.

Among the 29 patients with intact ventricular septum (IVS) there were six deaths (21% mortality), five in patients more than 12 months of age. Surgical mortality was 20% in patients who weighed more than 20 pounds (compared to 36% in smaller infants).

## Atrial Septectomy (Blalock-Hanlon Procedure)

For more than two decades atrial septectomy has been used as the procedure of choice as early surgical palliation of TGA. Only since September 1967 has BAS been used for initial palliation and thus the results in Table III reflect a transition in methods of treatment selection. Among 264 palliative operations, 207 included an atrial septectomy. In 132 patients, atrial septectomy alone was performed and in 75 atrial septectomy was done in combination with other palliative procedures including pulmonary systemic artery shunt and pulmonary banding. The operative mortality in the entire series of 264 patients was 26.5% and for atrial septectomy alone was 29.6%. Obviously many of the small infants arrived in the operating room in a moribund condition but all were included in this series even if the technical procedure was concluded just before death.

Table II. Operative Mortality of Mustard Procedure Related to Age and Weight (from Gutgesell & McNamara (16))

| Age (Months) | No. of Patients | No. of Deaths | Mortality (%) |
|---|---|---|---|
| 6 or less | 1 | 1 | 100 |
| 7–12 | 1 | 1 | 100 |
| 13–18 | 5 | 1 | 20 |
| 19–24 | 13 | 5 | 38 |
| 25–30 | 5 | | |
| Over 30 | 6 | | |
| | 31 | 8 | Overall 26% |
| Weight (pounds) | | | |
| 15 or less | 1 | 1 | 100 |
| 15–20 | 10 | 3 | 30 |
| 21–25 | 14 | 3 | 21 |
| Over 25 | 6 | 1 | 17 |
| | 31 | 8 | Overall 26% |

## Mustard Procedure

During the 10-year period during which we have performed the Mustard procedure as a definitive treatment for TGA, 182 patients underwent this procedure with 47 deaths (25.8%) (Table IV). Primary repair was performed in 67 patients (no previous palliative procedure) with 26 deaths (38.8%). This mortality was higher than that for any group of patients having undergone a previous palliative procedure.

Between April 1972 and July 1973 a contoured Dacron baffle was used as the patch material for the Mustard operation in 32 patients ranging in ages from seven weeks to eight years with a mean age of 2.8 years (8). Five patients were less than 12 months old and 12 were between 1 and 2 years. Seventeen patients were under 2 years and most weighed between 21 and 30 pounds (range 8 to 68 pounds). Of the 32 patients, 6 died in the 30-day postoperative period. In only one patient was caval obstruction suspected as a contributing cause of death. Of the 24 survivors, 8 required reoperation and in 7 the indication for reoperation was pulmonary venous obstruction (PVO). All seven of the reoperations were successful. Six patients had evidence of mild superior or inferior vena caval obstruction but none required reoperation for that indication. Reoperation for PVO was done from 6 to 17 months after the Mustard procedure and mean

Table III. Palliative Operations for Transposition of the Great Arteries (to Sept. 30, 1974)

| Procedure | Total | Early Deaths | Late Deaths | Early Deaths After Complete Repair | Late Deaths After Complete Repair |
|---|---|---|---|---|---|
| Creation of ASD[a] | 132 | 39 (29.6%) | 12 ( 9.1%) | | |
| Creation of ASD & PA[a] shunt | 35 | 7 (20.0%) | 5 (14.3%) | | |
| Creation of ASD, PA shunt and 2nd shunt | 2 | | | | |
| Creation of ASD at one op[a] and PA shunt at 2nd op | 9 | 2 (22.2%) [2nd op] | 1 (11.1%) | | |
| Creation of ASD and PA banding | 29 | 4 (13.8%) | | | |
| PA shunt | 42 | 12 (28.6%) | 4 ( 9.5%) | | |
| PA banding | 15 | 6 (40.0%) | 2 (13.3%) | | |
| Total | 264 | 70 (26.5%) | 24 ( 9.1%) | | |

[a]ASD = atrial septal defect; PA = pulmonary artery; op = operation.

Table IV. Mustard Procedures for Transposition of the Great Arteries (to Aug. 31, 1974)

| Procedure | No. of Patients | Early Deaths | Early Mortality Rate (%) |
|---|---|---|---|
| Mustard procedure | 182 | 47 | 25.8 |
| Previous Blalock-Hanlon | 68 | 13 | 19.1 |
| Previous Blalock-Hanlon and other palliative op[a] | 17 | 2 | 11.8 |
| Previous Rashkind (BAS)[a] | 18 | 1 | 5.6 |
| Other palliative op | 12 | 5 | 41.7 |
| Primary repair | 67 | 26 | 38.8 |

[a]op = operation; BAS = balloon atrial septostomy

reoperation time was 1 year. The occurrence of PVO was late in all patients and was not evident in the early postoperative course. As a result of the complications with the contoured Dacron baffle, autologous pericardium has been used in all operations performed subsequent to July 1973.

## DISCUSSION

A plan for management of newborn patients with TGA has evolved from our experience and may be at variance with other centers. While the risk of palliative and corrective procedures seems high, when compared to patients receiving no treatment whatsoever, the results are good. Previous studies by Liebman et al. (17) and Campbell (18) described first-year mortality approaching 90% before present methods of treatment were available. Kidd et al. (19) found a 95% mortality by age 2 years among patients with TGA before 1963.

The first 3 months of life is the period of greatest risk for the patient with TGA. Mortality in our patients within 1 week of BAS was 11% and within the first 3 months of life was 16%. The 3-month survival rate of 84% is an improvement over the survival rate of 25% before BAS was introduced (17).

In the past, palliative operations in patients with TGA were associated with a formidable mortality. For the Blalock-Hanlon procedure alone, reported mortalities range from 22 to 57% (20–23). At our institution, the mortality for palliative operation in patients with TGA was 30% before the introduction of BAS, but in the recent series of 32 atrial septectomies, the mortality was 9%. There were no deaths among patients over 2 months of age. The improved survival rate is most likely because the patients in this series were older and in better condition at the time of operation; in the earlier study many of the patients were critically ill, and 80% were under 3 months of age.

The overall results of the Mustard procedure were in general accord with other large series (24–26). Our recent experience suggests that intra-atrial baffle repair can be performed in cases of TGA without VSD or pulmonary hypertension with a mortality of less than 10% and in patients with VSD and moderate pulmonary hypertension, of approximately 15%.

In the past few years, some investigators have advocated a major change in the management of TGA: namely, abandoning most palliative operations and performing elective Mustard procedures in the 1st year of life (25, 27–30). Indeed, their early operative results have been very encouraging. Before adopting such a policy on a large scale, however, it is important to recognize that the consequences of TGA do not stop at the time of baffle repair. The problems of pulmonary vein and caval obstruction, arrhythmias, tricuspid insufficiency, and posthypothermia central nervous system disturbances are well known, and there is at least some indication that such problems may be more common when the procedure is performed on very small infants.

Champsaur et al. (26) reviewed the first 123 cases of baffle repair in Toronto and found a late death rate of 20% in the first 5 postoperative years. Breckenridge (25) reported a late mortality of 8.5% for 200 cases of Mustard procedure. Our late survival studies are similar. Thus, the survival rate after Mustard repair does not plateau with time but continues to decrease at a variable rate. Whether this rate is greater if the procedure is performed in the 1st year of life cannot be determined from the data presently available.

In view of our good results with palliative surgery and the relatively low mortality rate between the neonatal period and 1 year of age, we still prefer to defer the Mustard procedure to at least 12 months of age in cases of simple TGA. However, the slow weight gain between 12 and 24 months of age plus the development of pulmonary vascular obstructive disease in some patients prior to 24 months of age suggests there is little advantage, and perhaps some risk, in waiting to even 18 months.

Our management of patients with mild or moderate PS is similar to that of simple TGA; patients with severe PS are treated with systemic to pulmonary anastomosis and later correction. We still perform early banding and late correction for TGA with VSD.

## SUMMARY

Recent development in palliative and curative treatment of transposition of the great arteries have significantly improved the prognosis for this anomaly. All investigators now agree that early diagnosis within the first few days or weeks of life is necessary for optimum treatment and maximum survival. The balloon atrial septostomy provides a safe means of temporizing in the smallest infant, but more definitive measures must often be applied before the infant reaches 1 year of age.

While others have recently advocated an aggressive attack upon the anomaly during the neonatal period using hypothermic surgical techniques, our experience with a more conservative approach appears to provide a safer course with perhaps better late results. After balloon septostomy, we may use atrial septectomy (Blalock-Hanlon) combined often with pulmonary artery banding as a palliative second procedure. When the patient has attained an age of more than 18 months and weight of 24 pounds of more, the Mustard procedure using a pericardial atrial baffle may be employed with greater safety and better long-term prognosis. Alternative procedures to the Mustard technique are being employed in unusual cases of TGA associated with a large VSD.

## REFERENCES

1. Hanlon, C. R. and Blalock, A. 1945. Complete transposition of aorta and pulmonary artery: Experimental observations on venous shunts as corrective procedures. Ann. Surg. 127: 385.
2. Ochsner, J. L., Cooley, D. A., Harris, L. C., and McNamara, D. G. 1961. Treatment of complete transposition of great vessels with the Blalock-Hanlon operation. Circulation 24: 51.
3. Cooley, D. A. and Hallman, G. L. 1964. Surgery during the first year of life for cardiovascular anomalies: A review of 500 conservative operations. J. Cardiovasc. Surg. 5: 584.
4. Rashkind, W. K. and Miller, W. W. 1966. Creation of an atrial septal defect without thoracotomy: A palliative approach to complete transposition of the great vessels. JAMA 196: 991.
5. Albert, H. M. 1954. Surgical correction of transposition of great vessels. Surg. Forum 5: 74.
6. Mustard, W. T. 1964. Successful two-stage correction of transposition of the great vessels. Surgery 55: 419.
7. El-Said, G., Rosenberg, H. S., Mullins, C. E., Hallman, G. L., Cooley, D. A., and McNamara, D. G. 1972. Dysrhythmias after Mustard's operation for transposition of the great arteries. Am. J. Cardiol. 30: 526.
8. Reul, G. J., Jr., Cooley, D. A., Sandiford, F. M., and Hallman, G. L.

1974. Complications following the contoured Dacron baffle in correction of transposition of the great arteries. Surgery 76: 946.
9. Cooley, D. A., Wukasch, D. C., and Sandiford, F. M. 1973. Contoured knitted Dacron baffle for repair of transposition of the great vessels. Ann. Thorac. Surg. 15: 640.
10. Brom, A. G. 1974. Quoted (ref. 13) by Stark, J., de Leval, M. R., Waterston, D. J., Graham G. R., and Bonham-Carter, R. E. Corrective surgery of transposition of the great arteries in the first year of life: Results in 63 infants. J. Thorac. Cardiovasc. Surg. 67: 673.
11. Rastelli, G. C., McGoon, D. C., and Wallace, R. B. 1969. Anatomic correction of transposition of the great arteries with ventricular septal defect and subpulmonary stenosis. J. Thorac. Cardiovasc. Surg. 58: 545.
12. McGoon, D. C. 1972. Intraventricular repair of transposition of the great arteries. J. Thorac. Cardiovasc. Surg. 64: 430.
13. Anagnostopoulos, C. E., Athanasuleas, C. L., and Arcilla, R. A. 1973. Toward a rational operation for transposition of the great arteries. Ann. Thorac. Surg. 16: 458.
14. Balderman, S. C., Athanasuleas, C. L., and Anagnostopoulos, C. E. 1974. Coronary artery anatomy in transposition of the great vessels in relation to anatomic surgical correction. J. Thorac. Cardiovasc. Surg. 67: 208.
15. Stansel, H. C. A new operation for d-loop transposition of the great vessels. Ann. Thorac. Surg. (In press).
16. Gutgesell, H. P. and McNamara, D. G. 1975. Transposition of the great arteries: Results of treatment with early palliation and late intracardiac repair. Circulation 51: 32.
17. Liebman, J., Cullum, L., and Belloc, N. 1969. Natural history of transposition of the great arteries: Anatomy and birth and death characteristics. Circulation 40: 237.
18. Campbell, M. 1973. Incidence of cardiac malformations at birth and later, and neonatal mortality. Br. Heart J. 35: 189.
19. Kidd, B. S. L., Tyrell, M. J., and Pickering, D. 1971. Transposition 1969. In Kidd, B. S. L. and Keith, J. D. (Eds.). The Natural History and Progress in Treatment of Congential Heart Defects, pp. 127–137. Charles C. Thomas, Springfield.
20. Aberdeen, E., Waterston, D. J., Carr, I., Graham, G., Bonham-Carter, R. E., and Subramanian, S. 1965. Successful "correction" of transposed great arteries by Mustard's operation. Lancet 1: 1233.
21. Venables, A. W. 1966. Complete transposition of the great vessels in infancy with reference to palliative surgery. Br. Heart J. 28: 335.
22. Cornell, W. P., Maxwell, R. E., Haller, J. A., and Sabiston, D. C. 1966. Results of the Blalock-Hanlon operation in 90 patients with transposition of the great vessels. J. Thorac. Cardiovasc. Surg. 52: 525.
23. Plauth, W. H. Jr., Nadas, A. S. Bernhard, W. F., and Cross, R. E. 1968. Transposition of the great arteries: Clinical and physiological observations of 74 patients treated by palliative surgery. Circulation 37: 316.
24. Danielson, G. K., Mair, D. D., Ongley, P. A., Wallace, R. B., and McGoon, D. C. 1971. Repair of transposition of the great arteries by transposition of the venous return. J. Thorac. Cardiovasc. Surg. 61: 96.
25. Breckenridge, I. M., Stark, J., Bonham-Carter, R. E., Oelert, H.,

Graham, G. R., and Waterston, D. J. 1972. Mustard's operation for transposition of the great arteries: Review of 200 cases. Lancet 1: 1140.
26. Champsaur, G. L., Sokol, D. M., Trusler, G. A., and Mustard, W. T. 1973. Repair of transposition of the great arteries in 123 patients: Early and long-term results. Circulation 47: 1032.
27. Neutze, J. M. and Clarkson, P. M. 1973. Transposition of the great arteries in infancy. *In* Barratt-Boyes, B. G., Neutze, J. M., Harris, E. A. (Eds.). Heart Disease in Infancy: Diagnosis and Surgical Treatment, p. 269. Williams & Wilkins Co., Baltimore.
28. Venugopal, P., Olsyowka, J., Wagner, H., Vlad, P., Lambert, E., and Subramanian, S. 1973. Early correction of congenital heart disease with surface-induced deep hypothermia and circulatory arrest. J. Thorac. Cardiovasc. Surg. 66: 375.
29. Kilman, J. W., Williams, T. E. Jr., Kakos, G. S., Craenen, J., and Hosier, D. M. 1973. Surgical correction of the transposition complex in infancy. J. Thorac. Cardiovasc. Surg. 66: 387.
30. Bonchek, L. I. and Starr, A. 1972. Total correction of transposition of the great arteries in infancy as initial surgical management. Ann. Thorac. Surg. 14: 376.

# 8
# Panel on Transposition

**Moderator**
R. L. Replogle, M.D.
**Panel Members**
D. A. Cooley, M.D., R. A. Arcilla, M.D.,
N. E. Shumway, M.D., and C. E. Anagnostopoulos, M.D.

**Dr. Replogle**: The experience in correction of transposed great arteries with ventricular septal defect in Mustard's procedure in infants under 6 months of age is not very good. However, pulmonary artery banding procedures seem to have late complications at the time of debanding. Dr. Cooley, do you have any long-term follow-up on the patients in whom atrial septectomy and pulmonary banding was done for transposition, followed by Mustard's operation at a later date? Was subpulmonic obstruction or valve incompetence present at second operation due to the band?

**Dr. Cooley**: There are many objections to banding of the pulmonary artery, whether in VSD or transposition. I am inclined to believe that in small infants with transposition and a VSD it is perhaps better to do a palliative procedure than to attempt a corrective one. The choice depends on what one considers acceptable mortality. Some argue that an initial mortality of 40% for total correction is acceptable. Our cardiologists and I feel that such high initial mortality is unacceptable. I prefer a live kitten to a dead lion.

**Dr. Replogle**: Our results utilizing hypothermia for correction of transposition with ventricular septal defect in infancy have not been satisfactory. Dr. Arcilla will you comment?

**Dr. Arcilla**: In an infant with transposition and a large VSD without pulmonic stenosis there is excessive pulmonary blood flow and even under the most rigorous medical therapy some type of surgery is required to reduce this flow. I agree that the logical approach at the present time appears to be pulmonary artery banding. It also minimizes the risk of pulmonary vascular obstruction which may compromise the results of later corrective surgery. We are quite concerned that pulmonary artery banding does indeed compromise growth of the vessel or even of the pulmonic orifice, and may lead to iatrogenic pulmonic stenosis.

**Dr. Shumway**: With the availability of the porcine heterograft and the conduit operation it is possible to close the VSD in transposition in such a way that the posterior ventricle shunts blood under this patch and out the aorta anteriorly. A ventriculotomy is then placed in the anterior ventricle and a valve containing graft placed from this ventricle to a point on the pulmonary artery distal to the stenosis.

A slight variant of this procedure is illustrated by the case of a 7-year-old who had previous banding of the pulmonary artery due to a Taussig-Bing-like transposition with VSD. In this instance we sutured one end of a tubular graft to the margin of the VSD and the other to the base of the aortic valve thus directing the flow from the left ventricle through the graft and out the aorta. In the final stage of repair, we divide the pulmonary artery distal to the point of stenosis from the band and connect this to the right ventricle by means of a valve-containing tubular graft. These are the new ways of dealing with the problem of ventricular septal defect in transposition. We prefer to see a small VSD with pulmonic stenosis before attempting a conduit procedure since the left ventricle will more likely be able to cope with the systemic circulation.

**Dr. Replogle**: I would like to raise the problem of transposition of the great vessels accompanied by pulmonary atresia since we are discussing complex cases. Dr. Cooley, are you involved in the atrial-pulmonary artery conduit procedure, the Fontain operation?

**Dr. Cooley**: I have not done the Fontain procedure for tricuspid atresia or other hypoplastic conditions. Presently, we employ palliative operations for tricuspid atresia. We must have skepticism about the long-term results of placing a Dacron graft containing a valve in such small patients. Too often what is called a corrective procedure is nothing more than radical palliation.

**Dr. Replogle**: Dr. Shumway, what do you tell the patients after a successful Mustard operation? Is the child cured?

**Dr. Shumway**: I do not think one should use the word "cured," but rather "corrected." The greatest danger is in the immediate postoperative period. If during this time there is no sign of obstruction of venous return to the heart, then there is a good chance the procedure was successful. With respect to the right ventricle and tricuspid valve, patients with corrected transposition live essentially normal lives with internal cardiac anatomy similar to that seen in the post-Mustard heart. Some such patients do require valve replacement later on. This apparently corrective procedure does allow for overall symptomatic improvement, and follow-up is essential. Perhaps one day the operation suggested by Dr. Anagnostopoulos, of directly switching the great vessels may become useful as we accumulate data on the results of present surgery for transposition, and as the newer experimental operations are refined.

**Dr. Replogle**: Dr. Anagnostopoulos, will you comment on your proposed new operation for transposition of the great arteries?

**Dr. Anagnostopoulos**: Mustard's operation carries the long-term complications of venous obstruction, tricuspid insufficiency, and dysrhythmia. Since the anatomy of the right ventricle and valve do not appear suited for a normal lifetime of systemic pumping, we have proposed a new operation which involves switching the aorta and pulmonary artery to restore normal anatomic continuity. Of course, the coronary arteries would need to be switched as well and this was the limiting feature of previous attempts at direct repair of transposition. It appears from our data, however, that the anatomy of the coronaries in transposition is favorable for such a procedure. The length of the coronary arteries until the first branch was measured and the distance the coronary ostium would need to be moved onto its new site on the proximal pulmonary artery was measured. Comparison of these values indicated that in most instances, if the coronary arteries are left on the aorta and an incision carried below the coronary ostia but above the valve, such a switch of aorta and pulmonary artery can be accomplished. We have done this procedure in the laboratory in an attempt to create an animal model of transposition with the aid of deep hypothermia, circulatory arrest, and microsurgical techniques. As the right ventricle is not prepared to pump systemically, survival has been, as expected, limited to a few hours. However, the feasibility of such an approach has been well demonstrated. The Mustard operation can today be accomplished with amazingly low mortality, 5% in some centers, and it is difficult to present a new operation for clinical trial which in its initial stages will carry a much higher mortality. Perhaps we should reserve this new operation for infants with transposition and VSD or those children who have grown into their teens and are not doing well with their Mustard operation. At that time the switch operation would be technically much simpler than on an infant. And if the coronary artery anatomy is not favorable, saphenous or arterial coronary bypass grafts could be employed. Of course there is the additional problem of preparing the left ventricle so that it will be able to pump systemically after the surgery. It would be easy to enter it via venous puncture since the venous circulation communicates directly with the left ventricle. Perhaps a catheter with an inflatable balloon tip could be placed in the ventricle, creating partial obstruction thereby stimulating a certain degree of ventricular hypertrophy.

**Dr. Replogle**: Thank you.

# Dissections III

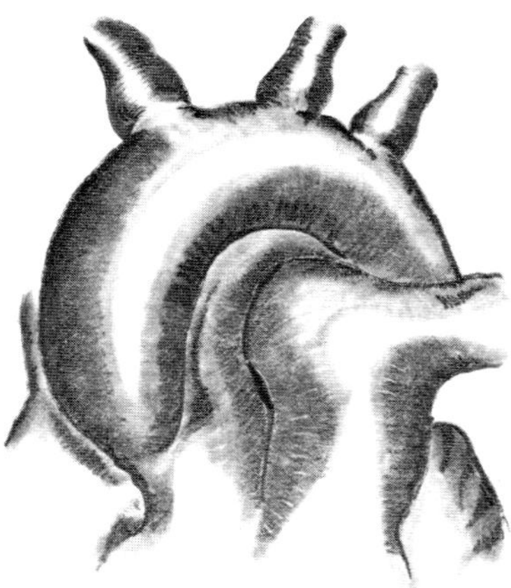

Acute Aortic Dissections:
Introduction and
Medical Therapy

The Aorta
in the Marfan Syndrome
and Other Genetic Disorders
of Connective Tissue

Surgical Therapy
of Dissection
of the Aorta

Cardiac Anesthesia
for Lethal Diseases of
the Ascending Aorta

Panel on
Acute Aortic Dissection

# 9 Acute Aortic Dissections: Introduction and Medical Therapy

C. L. Athanasuleas, M.D.,
C. E. Anagnostopoulos, M.D., and
L. Resnekov, M.D.

Though for the most part the management of acute aortic dissections is regarded as surgical, over the years indications have been accumulated which suggest temporary or prolonged medical therapy. The principles of such treatment are based on a sound understanding of the pathophysiology of the disease and are essential in the management of all patients with dissection, whether handled medically or surgically. Early intervention in acute aortic dissection is imperative.

This review deals with clinical aspects of dissection, the indications for medical therapy and its methods, and the results of such treatment.

The term "dissecting aneurysm" of the aorta is really a misnomer. Since in most instances the disease presents as an acute process there is no "aneurysm," but rather a dissecting hematoma. It is appropriate, therefore, that the disease be called "acute aortic dissection."

In the first few hours or days after dissection the chest x-ray may appear normal without obvious aortic dilatation. It is the most common lethal catastrophe of the aorta and without rapid intervention at the time of presentation may be followed by disastrous sequelae (1). In a review of untreated cases within the first 48 hr. of dissection 50% died and by the end of one year approximately 90% were no longer alive (2) (Fig. 1). From these data it is possible to extrapolate the prognosis of a patient who

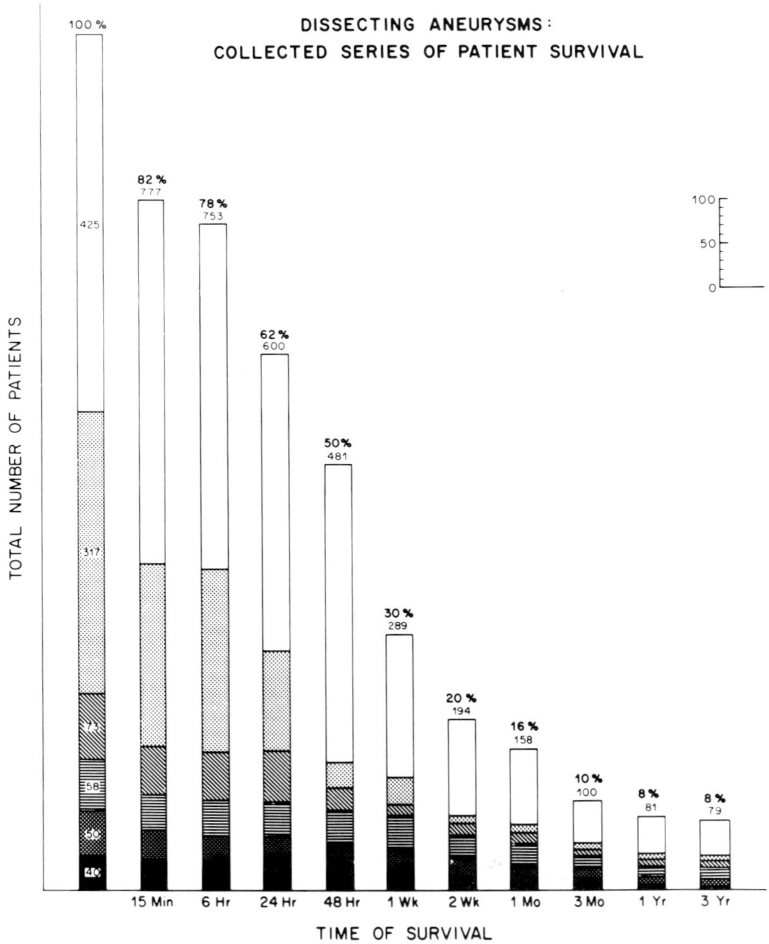


Figure 1. The fate of untreated aortic dissection and dissecting aneurysms. (Reprinted from *Acute Aortic Dissections* by C. E. Anagnostopoulos, University Park Press, Baltimore.)

presents with the classical findings of acute dissection (Table I). It is seen that a delay of only a few days may double the risk of death.

The usual patient with dissection of the aorta presents with acute pain, described variously as burning, tearing, or excruciating which may be felt in the anterior midchest, in the left chest, in the submental, substernal, facial, epigastric, or interscapular areas, as well as in the neck, midback, and sacral areas depending on the actual size and extension of the dissection (3). Neurological symptoms include headache, syncope, transient

Table I. The Prognosis of Untreated Dissection

| Time after the Onset of Symptoms | Risk of Death (%) |
|---|---|
| Less than 15 min. | 3 |
| 15 min. | 35 |
| 48 hr. | 36 |
| 1 week | 75 |
| 3 months | 89 |

blindness or paralysis and coma. Dyspnea and orthopnea are common cardiorespiratory symptoms and may reflect tracheal compression, hemothorax, acute cardiac failure from aortic regurgitation (20% of patients), or pericardial tamponade. Hemoptysis may result from dissection of the descending aorta into the hilum of the lung. If the involvement extends into the abdominal aorta, gastrointestinal dilatation due to ischemia may occur, resulting in nausea and vomiting. Hematemesis and melena are severe signs and carry a poor prognosis. Renal involvement may cause oliguria, hematuria, or anuria.

The physical findings often reveal the extent and severity of the dissecting process (2, 3). Cardiomegaly is present in about two-thirds of patients, probably secondary to their hypertensive disease. Bloody pleural and pericardial effusions may result from leakage through adventitial tears. The diastolic murmur of aortic regurgitation occurs in 25% of patients due to loss of commisural support. A duplication of pulses is the consequence of flow in the true as well as false lumen. If an intimal flap obstructs an arterial branch the pulse may disappear temporarily, intermittently, or permanently.

Laboratory investigations should include a blood count, blood urea nitrogen (BUN), creatinine, and amylase. In subacute and chronic forms of dissection, a normochromic normocytic anemia may be present as well as leucocytosis (3). The erythrocyte sedimentation rate is almost invariably elevated. Fibrinolysis may also occur due to release of subintimal tissue fibrinolysins (4). An elevated BUN and creatinine may be due to decreased renal perfusion or renal infarction secondary to direct renal artery involvement in the dissection. If the dissection involves the superior mesenteric artery with hemorrhage around the head of the pancreas, the serum amylase is usually increased.

The electrocardiographic abnormalities in dissection are not pathognomonic and ischemia or infarction patterns are seen in 10 to 30% of cases and 10% show pericarditis (3). Echocardiography sometimes demonstrates simultaneous pulsating echoes indicating the presence of a double lumen (5).

Posteroanterior and lateral projections in addition to the standard view may show the characteristic radiographic findings of superior mediastinal widening, widening of the distal aortic knob beyond the subclavian artery or a double shadow density. Occasionally the chest x-ray is normal. In rare cases of anterior (ascending aortic) dissection, in the presence of life-threatening complications surgery has been performed immediately, before angiograms could be obtained. In the presence of shock, hemopericardium, or hemothorax angiography in itself does not appear to carry increased risk. However, it is generally contraindicated in such instances since the progression of the disease is rapid and the delay required for such studies may result in increased mortality (6). In the usual case direct retrograde intra-arterial injection is performed and the intimal tear is seen as a radioluscent line. If the false lumen fills, a "double lumen" is seen and if the catheter is placed into the true lumen the major arterial branches will visualize.

It has long been suggested that the anatomic location of the dissection is a key factor in determining the type of therapy and prognosis. The original classification of DeBakey documented three types of dissection (7). In type I the intimal tear occurs at various sites in the ascending aorta and the dissecting hematoma may extend throughout the length of the aorta. In type II the dissection is limited to the ascending aorta, and in type III it occurs beyond the subclavian artery, thus limiting the process to the descending aorta. Since the prognosis of types I and II are known to be similar, Shumway and Austen have suggested a classification based on the fact that acute dissections involving the ascending aorta, "anterior lesions," are high risk and those involving the descending aorta, "posterior lesions," can be considered low risk (8, 9).

An important feature of aortic dissection, however, and one which has not been stressed in the classification offered thus far is the presence or absence of complications in addition to the anatomic site of the tear. We propose, therefore, the following classification (10). Class A dissections are those involving the ascending aorta, and class B dissections those which do not involve the ascending aorta. These types are subdivided further on the basis of the presence or absence of complications. Group 1 denotes complications such as shock, severe aorta regurgitation, saccular aneurysm, intrapericardial bleeding, myocardial ischemia, sudden onset of right bundle branch block, reversible neurological signs of carotid artery obstruction, pulmonary artery obstruction, impending rupture on x-ray or renal involvement. Included also are the specific diagnostic findings of Marfan's disease, coarctation of the aorta, as well as the special circumstance of pregnancy. Group 2 dissections have none of the complications listed above. Finally, class C dissections are those occurring in a patient who is inoperable due to the presence of another life-threatening disease such as cancer. The exact anatomy of the lesion is often unknown since many of these patients do not undergo complete diagnostic evaluation.

The indications for surgical or medical therapy depend on the classification of dissection at the time of admission (Table II). Class $A_1$ dissections require emergency surgery and early surgery is indicated for class $A_2$. If the intimal tear occurs in the descending aorta with complications (class $B_1$), medical therapy is recommended followed by surgery as soon as possible. Class B dissections without complications ($B_2$) may be handled by medical therapy alone, particularly if the patient's condition is stable even in the presence of untreated hypertension.

A classification based on the etiology of the disease has not been developed. It is known that certain other conditions predispose to dissection (10). These include Marfan's disease, Erdheim's medial cystic necrosis, giant cell aortitis, coarctation of the aorta, and pregnancy. Experimentally lathyrism, epinepherine excess, and copper deficiency have been shown to cause lesions of the intima with the formation of a dissecting hematoma. The duration of dissection is yet another variable into which a particular dissection could be classified. However, the simple distinction of anatomic site seems to be the most influential determinant of therapy.

Medical therapy is based on the observation that rupture of the aorta in some strains of turkeys could be prevented if their hypertension was controlled by reserpine (11). It was subsequently shown that dissection can be controlled also by reducing myocardial contractile force during systole (12–18). Thus medical management is designed to lower blood pressure and to reduce myocardial contractility by the use of beta adrenergic blocking agents.

Table II. New "ABC" Treatment Classification of Dissections

| Class | Treatment |
|---|---|
| A. Involve ascending aorta | |
| $A_1$ with complications | Medical, earliest surgery |
| $A_2$ without complications | Medical, planned surgery |
| B. Do not involve ascending aorta | |
| $B_1$ with complications | Medical, early surgery |
| $B_2$ without complications | Medical, ? elective surgery |
| C. Inoperable | Medical |

The indications for medical therapy are:
1. *A clotted false lumen* (17). In such cases the clot is thought to protect the aorta from the progression of the dissecting process. It is important that this be distinguished from failure to visualize the false lumen at the time of angiography. Multiple angiographic views are necessary before it is concluded that the lumen is clotted.
2. *The absence of a distinct site of the aortic intimal tear on angiography, in the absence of complicating features.*
3. *Dissection involving the ascending or descending aorta not accompanied by acute complications.* Since acute survival in class $A_2$ dissections is the same among medically and surgically treated groups (19), a case can be made for temporary medical therapy but only if the ascending dissection is uncomplicated. Such patients are at risk of immediate death and amenable to non-surgical care early in the disease. Therapy consisting of control of previously untreated hypertension is an important contribution in the care of both class $A_2$ and $B_2$ dissections and may be all that is required.
4. *Stable redissection.* Although it might appear that in cases of redissection medical therapy alone would be insufficient, the results of a survey we carried out indicate that no difference exists between redissections treated medically and those treated surgically (19).
5. *The presence of multiple intimal tears.* Tears may be present in the ascending, descending, and abdominal aortas. Although this precludes total repair in one operation, such patients may benefit by surgical procedures done in stages. In a patient described by Cooley four sequential operations were needed to replace almost the entire aorta (20)! The segment of aorta which contains life-threatening tears should be replaced even in the presence of other tears.
6. *Unavailable surgical facilities, or patient refusal to undergo surgery.* Under these circumstances vigorous medical therapy is essential and the level of blood pressure should be reduced rapidly in a monitored setting.

## MEDICAL THERAPY

As stressed earlier, the principle of medical therapy is the control of the blood pressure and a reduction in the force of myocardial contraction. The following regimen, which is based on our own experience, is recommended. On suspicion and throughout investigative tests blood pressure must be carefully monitored. The patient is placed in an intensive care unit and the appropriate catheters are inserted to monitor continually arterial and venous pressure. Heart rate and urine output should also be carefully followed. Serial electrocardiograms and serum enzyme determinations (CPK, SGOT, SGPT) are obtained. The blood pressure is maintained at about 110/70 using trimethaphan (Arfonad), 500 mg. in 500 ml. 5% dextrose and water beginning at a rate of 50 mcgm./kg./min. and regulated according to blood pressure response. Tachyphylaxis may develop within 1 or 2 days. Sodium nitroprusside may be substituted for trimethaphan, 50 mg. being diluted in 500 ml. 5% dextrose and water and administered intravenously in a dose of 0.3 to 60 mcgm./kg./min. Careful monitoring of blood pressure and heart rate is essential and any major side effects should be managed by slowing the rate of infusion. If these agents are ineffective in the management of the hypertension, diazoxide (Hyperstat) may be administered as a bolus of 300 mg. intravenously.

By the 2nd to 5th day of medical therapy methyldopa (Aldomet), 250 to 500 mg. every four hours i.v. or p.o. or guanethidine, 25 mg. p.o. t.i.d. may be substituted. If the patient is not being stabilized for immediate surgery, propranolol in doses of 20 to 40 mg. four times daily is given by mouth. A heart rate of approximately 60 is desired.

Assuming the patient continues pain-free and vital signs remain normal, he may be moved within 1 week to a non-intensive care setting and arm cuff blood pressure measured every 2 hours.

In uncomplicated cases the patient may be discharged within 2 weeks of admission if hypertension is under control. A chronic regimen of antihypertensives as well as oral propranolol 20 to 40 mg. is maintained after discharge and the patient is instructed to visit the clinic or office at intervals of 2 weeks, 1 month, and then at 3-month intervals for 1 year. Thereafter, he may be seen twice yearly.

Frequent visits are necessary, since localized saccular aneurysms develop in about 15% of class B patients treated by pharmacologic means alone. And among class A patients treated medically, 10% will ultimately require aortic valve replacement due to progressive regurgitation (15). It is important that chest x-rays be obtained on each visit, as cardiac enlargement or the development of saccular aneurysm may necessitate further study by means of angiography. An aortogram is the best means of assessing the patient's status and should be routinely performed 1 year after the initial hospitalization. Finally, the patient should be educated that chest or back pain in the case of previous class A aortic dissection, or abdominal pain following a class B dissection may be a grave prognostic sign and that he should immediately alert his physician if it should occur. Table III summarizes the various subclasses of dissection and indicates the recommended form of therapy on a time scale.

Table III. Therapy of Acute Dissection According to Site and Presenting Features

| Class | General Operability | Presentation | Rx 0–4 hr. | Rx 4–24 hr. | Rx 1–4 weeks | Rx After 1 month |
|---|---|---|---|---|---|---|
| $A_1$ | Yes | Complicated[a] | Drugs | Surgery | Drugs | Drugs |
| $A_2$ | Yes | Uncomplicated | Drugs | Drugs | Drugs → Surgery | Drugs |
| $B_1$ | Yes | Complicated[a] | Drugs | Surgery | Drugs | Drugs |
| $B_2$[b] | Yes | Uncomplicated | Drugs | Drugs | Drugs<br>? Surgery | Drugs<br>? Surgery |
| C | No | Complicated[a] or Uncomplicated | | | | |

[a]Resistant shock, overwhelming aortic insufficiency, saccular aneurysm, tamponade, myocardial ischemia, reversible central nervous system signs, pulmonary artery obstruction, right bundle branch block, resistance to antihypertensives, impending rupture radiographically, renal obstruction, carotid obstruction, absence of hypertension, and the conditions of Marfan's disease or pregnancy. [a] = *one or more of these.*

[b]Includes all clotted false lumens.

## RESULTS OF TREATMENT

The results of therapy in recent years have demonstrated the effectiveness of medical management in certain instances and elucidated the role of surgical management. Thus Wheat reported a 62% survival 1 to 3 years after the acute event among 64 patients treated medically, but of the living patients, 25% eventually required surgery (13). In 1972, McFarland et al. emphasized the prognostic difference between lesions of the ascending and descending aorta. Six patients with ascending aortic dissection were treated medically and two survived whereas there were only six deaths up to 2½ years among 25 patients with this lesion treated surgically (17, 21). Descending aortic dissections carried a better prognosis and eight of ten patients treated medically survived up to 43 months.

In a recent survey (19), Athanasuleas and Anagnostopoulos collected 280 cases of aortic dissection from the literature and 269 cases from questionnaires sent to major medical centers in the United States and abroad to obtain a 30-day survival and the late results up to 5 years after the acute event, and these data are summarized in Table IV. A comparison of subgroups was carried out and Student's t-test applied to determine statistical significance. With respect to class A dissections, it is noted in Table V that acute survival appears to be greater among the medically treated group (77% versus 68%), but this difference is not significant ($p > 0.25$). However, chronic survival, that is survival to 5 years, is better among class A patients treated surgically.

In contrast, in class B dissections there is no statistical difference in the acute or chronic groups treated medically or surgically. Patients in this group (class $B_2$) should therefore be managed medically and observed carefully for the development of complications which might indicate the need for surgical intervention.

## SUMMARY

Acute aortic dissection is a lethal disease and must be treated immediately on presentation. Physical findings are often a clue to the anatomic site of the dissection and angiography serves to confirm it. Surgical therapy of acute dissection is indicated if it involves the ascending aorta (class A) and in those cases not involving the ascending aorta (class B) if the patient presents with either Marfan's syndrome, pregnancy, or coarctation of the aorta (class $A_1$). Surgery is also indicated in the presence of complications which include 1) resistant shock, 2) overwhelming aortic regurgitation, 3) saccular aneurysm, 4) pericardial bleeding, 5) myocardial ischemia, 6)

Table IV. Survival in Aortic Dissections

| | Class A | Class B | A & B |
|---|---|---|---|
| Surgery | | | |
| Acute survival (literature) | 74/109 = 68% | 70/106 = 66% | |
| Chronic survival (questionnaire) | 78/110 = 71% | 54/90 = 60% | |
| Redissections (questionnaire) | 10/110 = 9% | 2/90 = 2% | |
| Medicine | | | |
| Acute survival (literature) | 24/31 = 77% | 28/34 = 82% | |
| Chronic survival (questionnaire) | 20/40 = 50% | 22/29 = 76% | |
| Redissections (questionnaire) | 5/40 = 12% | 1/29 = 3% | |
| Total redissections (questionnaire) medical and surgical | 15/150 = 10% | 3/119 = 3% | 18/269 = 7% |
| Redissections (literature and questionnaire) medical and surgical | | | 62/549 = 11% |
| Total no. of patients from literature review | | | 280 |
| Total no. of patients from questionnaire | | | 269 |
| Total | | | 549 |

Table V. Statistical Comparison of Subgroups

| Survival and Mode of Therapy | Significant Difference at 95% Confidence Level ($p < 0.05$) |
|---|---|
| Class A acute: surgery (68%) versus medicine (77%) | No |
| Class A chronic: surgery (71%) versus medicine (50%) | Yes |
| Class A redissection: surgery (9%) versus medicine (12%) | No |
| Class B acute: surgery (66%) versus medicine (82%) | No |
| Class B chronic: surgery (60%) versus medicine (76%) | No |
| Class B redissection: surgery (2%) versus medicine (3%) | No |
| Redissection, surgery + medicine: A (10%) versus B (3%) | No |

Table VI. Results of Therapy at The University of Chicago[a]

| Type | No. of Cases | Treatment | | 30-Day Survival | | Late Survival | |
|---|---|---|---|---|---|---|---|
| | | Medical | Surgical | Medical | Surgical | Medical | Surgical |
| Type I (class A) | 8 | 1 | 7 | 1/1 | 5/7 | 1/1 | 4/7 |
| Type II (class A) | 9 | 1 | 8 | 1/1 | 7/8 | 1/1 | 6/8 |
| Total I and II (class A) | 17 | 1 | 15 | 2/2 | 12/15 | 2/2 | 10/15 |
| Type III (class B) | 19 | 7 | 12 | 4/7 | 9/12 | 4/7 | 7/12 |
| Total | 36 | 9 | 27 | 6/9 | 21/27 | 6/9 | 17/27 |

[a]Reprinted from *Acute Aortic Dissections* by C. E. Anagnostopoulos, University Park Press, Baltimore.

Table VII. Improved Survival since Prospective Treatment Protocol Based on New "ABC" Classification[a]

| | | Treatment | | 30-Day Survival | | Late Survival | |
|---|---|---|---|---|---|---|---|
| Class | No. of Patients | Medical | Surgical | Medical | Surgical | Medical | Surgical |
| $A_1$ | 11 | | 11 | N.A.[b] | 10/11 (91%) | N.A. | 8/11 (73%) |
| $A_2$ | 3 | 3 | | 3 | N.A. | 3[c]/3 | N.A. |
| $B_1$ | 3 | | 3 | N.A. | 3/3 | N.A. | 3/3 |
| $B_2$ | 3 | 3 | | 3/3 | N.A. | 3/3 | N.A. |
| Total | 20 | 6 | 14 | 6/6 (100%) | 13/14 (93%) | 6[c]/6 (100%) | 11/14 (79%) |

[a]Reprinted from *Acute Aortic Dissections* by C. E. Anagnostopoulos, University Park Press, Baltimore.
[b]Not applicable.
[c]One patient may require surgery.

reversible central nervous system signs, 7) pulmonary artery obstruction, 8) sudden onset of right bundle branch block, 9) resistance to antihypertensives, and 10) impending signs of rupture radiographically (class $A_1$). Medical therapy is best applied if 1) there is a clotted false lumen, 2) an unidentifiable site of intimal tear, 3) either a class A or B dissection unaccompanied by the complications listed above (classes $A_2$ and $B_2$), 4) stable redissection, 5) multiple intimal tears, and 6) unavailable facilities or patient refusal.

The importance of the accurate localization and extent of the dissection is stressed and the need for careful monitoring in an intensive care unit during the acute stage indicated. Thereafter progressive care is maintained with adequate blood pressure control and after discharge from the hospital the patient should be seen at routine intervals with sequential chest x-rays and electrocardiograms to confirm a stable situation and plan effectively for future management. The experience at the University of Chicago (Tables VI and VII) reflects improved results utilizing strict adherence to the new classification.

## REFERENCES


1. Sorensen, H. R. and Olsen, H. 1964. Ruptured and dissecting aneurysms of the aorta. Incidence and prospects of surgery. Acta Chir. Scand. 128: 644.
2. Anagnostopoulos, C. E., Prabhakar, M. J. S., and Kittle, C. F. 1972. Aortic dissections and dissecting aneurysms. Am. J. Cardiol. 30: 263–273.
3. Levinson, D. C., Edmeades, D. T., and Griffith, G. C. 1950. Dissecting aneurysm of the aorta: its clinical, electrocardiographic and laboratory features; report of fifty eight autopsied cases. Circulation 1: 360.
4. Sendler, G. P. 1973. Aneurysm dissequant de l'ante responsible d'une coagulopathie d'consummation. Presse Nouvelle Med. 2: 971.
5. Nanda, N. C., Gramiak, R., and Shah, P. M. 1973. Diagnosis of aortic root dissection by echocardiography. Circulation 48: 506.
6. Soto, B., Harman, M. A., Ceballos, R., and Barcia, A. 1972. Angiographic diagnosis of dissecting aneurysm of the aorta. Am. J. Roentgenol. 116: 146.
7. DeBakey, M. D., Cooley, D. A., and Creech, O., Jr. 1955. Surgical consideration of dissecting aneurysm of the aorta. Ann. Surg. 142: 586.
8. Austen, W. G., Buckley, M. J., and McFarland, J. 1969. Therapeutic approach for dissecting aneurysm. Bull. Soc. Internatl. Surg. 28: 261.
9. Daily, P. O., Trueblood, H. W., Stinson, E. B., Wuerflein, R. D., and Shumway, N. E. 1970. Management of acute aortic dissections. Ann. Thor. Surg. 10: 237.
10. Anagnostopoulos, C. E. 1975. Acute Aortic Dissections. University Park Press, Baltimore.

11. McSherry, B. J., Ferguson, A. E., and Ballantyne, J. 1954. Dissecting aneurysm and internal hemorrhage in turkeys. J. Am Vet. Med. Assoc. 124: 279–283.
12. Wheat, M. W., Jr., Palmer, R. F., Bartley, T. D., and Seelman, R. C. 1965. Treatment of dissecting aneurysms of the aorta without surgery. J. Thor. Cardiovasc. Surg. 50: 364.
13. Wheat, M. W., Jr. and Palmer, R. F. 1969. Acute dissecting aneurysms of the aorta: Treatment and results in 64 patients. J. Thor. Cardiovasc. Surg. 58: 344.
14. Lindsay, J. and Hurst, J. W.: Drug therapy of dissecting aortic aneurysms. Some reservations. Circulation 37: 216.
15. Wheat, M. W. 1973. Treatment of dissecting aneurysms. A review. Progr. Cardiovasc. Dis. 16: 87–101.
16. Wheat, M. W., Jr. and Palmer, R. F. 1971. Dissecting aneurysms of the aorta. Current Problems in Surgery. New York Medical Publishers Inc., Chicago.
17. McFarland, J., Willerson, J. T., Dinsmore, R. E., Austen, W. G., Buckley, M. J., Sanders, C. A., and DeSanctis, R. W. 1972. The medical treatment of dissecting aortic aneurysms. N. Engl. J. Med. 286: 115.
18. Prokop, E. K., Palmer, R. F., and Wheat, M. W., Jr. 1970. Hydrodynamic forces in dissecting aneurysms. In vitro studies in a Tygon model and in dog aortas. Circ. Res. 27: 121.
19. Athanasuleas, C. L. 1975. The treatment of acute aortic dissections: A statistical analysis. *In* Acute Aortic Dissections, by C. E. Anagnostopoulos. University Park Press, Baltimore.
20. Cooley, D. A. Preceding chapter. Panel discussion on acute aortic dissection.
21. Austen, W. G. 1971. Comment in paper by Liotta, D., Hallman, G. L., Milam, J. D., et al. Surgical treatment of acute intramural dissection of the ascending aorta. Ann. Thorac. Surg. 12: 582.

# 10 The Aorta in the Marfan Syndrome and Other Genetic Disorders of Connective Tissue

V. A. McKusick, M.D.

The heritable disorders of connective tissue may be classified into those in which the basic lesion appears to occur in the fibrous components and those in which the mucopolysaccharide is the main site of involvement, e.g., the Hurler syndrome. Examples of the former category (to which this discussion will be limited) include the Marfan syndrome, the Ehlers-Danlos syndromes and osteogenesis imperfecta. Some progress has been made in understanding the nature of the molecular defect in several forms of the Ehlers-Danlos syndrome and one form of osteogenesis imperfecta, but such is not the case with the Marfan syndrome.

In its full manifestation the Marfan syndrome is characterized by eye involvement, especially subluxation of the lenses, but also myopia and retinal detachment; by skeletal features, which include loosejointedness and excessive limb length (called in the case of the fingers arachnodactyly); and by cardiovascular lesions such as diffuse aortic aneurysm or dissection of the aorta. The mitral valve may be involved as well, leading to mitral regurgitation, a conspicuous finding in some patients.

The Marfan syndrome is inherited as an autosomal dominant trait. Its manifestations result from a single mutant gene. Because variability is a rule in genetic diseases (as it indeed is in all disease), it is not surprising to find different features of the disease in affected persons even within the same family. The principles of medical genetics well illustrated by the Marfan syndrome are mainly three: 1) pleiotropism, which means multiple clinical effects of a single gene, 2) variability, and 3) genetic heterogeneity, i.e., what may appear to be a single gene-determined condition is actually more than one, each determined by separate genetic or environmental causes.

Figure 3–24 in *Heritable Disorders of Connective Tissue* (1) illustrates the variability which can exist in the Marfan syndrome, even within the same family. The father of the brothers shown died of the Marfan syndrome at 35 years of age. The younger brother had dislocated lenses, and severe skeletal features with spinal curvature. The older brother was tall, with scoliosis. However, eye examination showed no dislocated lenses or other significant abnormality. The younger brother had considerable mitral regurgitation, whereas the older brother had an acute aortic dissection which required replacement of the aortic valve and ascending aorta about 11 years after this picture was taken. Such variation in the manifestation of the Marfan syndrome within the family is a result of differences in the gene background against which the single major gene operates.

Genetic heterogeneity means that the Marfan syndrome may occur in different forms, or that fundamentally distinct disorders share certain features so that they are considered in the same category. About 10 years ago homocystinuria, which demonstrates many of the clinical features of the Marfan syndrome, was recognized as a separate entity and its biochemical lesion elucidated. Suffice it to say that, although the lenses are dislocated in homocystinuria (usually downward as an acquired feature occurring in the first or second decade of life rather than the upward dislocation of the lens present already at birth as in the Marfan syndrome) and although the skeletal features in severe cases may be rather similar to those in the Marfan syndrome, aortic involvement of the type seen in the Marfan syndrome does not occur, nor does mitral valve involvement. Thrombosis, either arterial or venous, is the main cardiovascular complication of homocystinuria.

As knowledge is accumulated at the clinical and biochemical level, sub-classes of the Marfan syndrome are likely to emerge. Already several seemingly distinct forms can be recognized on clinical grounds. In infants and children, for example, an *asthenic* form is recognized by the occurrence of markedly loose joints, underdevelopment of skeletal musculature and often severe mitral valve involvement. Survival beyond age 15 years is uncommon in these cases. (See Figures 3-23 and 3-29 in my *Heritable*

*Disorders of Connective Tissue,* 1972, for examples.) Other children, as well as adults, are *non-asthenic*. They are very tall, often with dislocated lenses and seem to have a particular propensity to develop aortic aneurysm and aortic dissection, although aortic problems develop in the asthenic form also. (See Figure 3-56 in *Heritable Disorders of Connective Tissue* (1) for an example of the non-asthenic form.)

A third group of Marfan patients shows stretchable skin and exceedingly hypermobile joints, features particularly common in the Ehlers-Danlos syndrome. They are tall, often with severe pectus excavatum, and have aortic dilatation. This has been called the *Marfanoid hypermobility syndrome*. (See Figure 3-71 in *Heritable Disorders of Connective Tissues,* for an example. In the last 2 years the patient has developed aortic regurgitation and dilatation of the first part of the aorta demonstrable by echogram.)

Yet a fourth form of the Marfan syndrome has been known in recent years as *contractural arachnodactyly*. It is probably the disorder present in the patient Marfan described in Paris in 1896. Aortic and other cardiovascular involvement has not yet been described, to my knowledge, in contractual arachnodactyly.

Most frequently the aortic changes in the Marfan syndrome involve the ascending aorta in which progressive dilatation begins sometimes in the 1st year or so of life, sometimes not until the 4th or 5th decade, or even later. At some point thereafter dissection may take place in the aorta, the intimal rent most often occurring in the ascending aorta. The progressive dilation of the ascending aorta involves first the intrapericardial portions. As a result, aortic regurgitation producing a diastolic murmur is often the first manifestation of the onset of this process and may precede signs by ordinary radiographic techniques. Contrast aortography provides definitive demonstration of dilatation, of course, and in recent times the non-invasive technique of echocardiography has been exceedingly useful in detecting the presence and progression of dilatation in the ascending aorta. The normal dimensions of the aorta by echocardiogram, for various ages and body sizes, are in the process of being determined.

We believe that dissection of the aorta in the Marfan syndrome rarely occurs completely "out of the blue." Patients usually, if not always, have pre-existing dilatation in the aorta. Hence patients should be watched closely for the development of aortic dilatation as indicated by the murmur of aortic regurgitation or of the dilatation of the aorta by radiography or echocardiography. It is our practice to follow-up patients with the Marfan syndrome at least annually.

Dissections are classified by DeBakey into type I, if they involve the entire aorta with rent beginning in the ascending aorta; type II, if their origin and extent are limited to the ascending aorta; and type III, if they occur beyond the subclavian arterial ostium involving the descending thoracic and abdominal aorta. Examples of all three types of dissections have been observed in the Marfan syndrome, but the most frequent form is type II.

Survivorship in the Marfan syndrome has been studied by the life-table method (see Figure 3-54 in *Heritable Disorders of Connective Tissue*). Between ages 30 and 55 years, males fare less well than females. Probability of survival to age 60 years was found to be about 30% for both male and female Marfan patients, as compared with values of about 80% and 90% for males and females in the general population. Data such as these must be interpreted in light of the strong probability that the Marfan syndrome as we know it today is a lumping of several fundamentally distinct entities.

The medical management of the aortic problem of the Marfan syndrome makes use of propranolol on a long-term basis. The beta-adrenergic blocking agent reduces the abruptness of ventricular ejection, thereby reducing the physiologic trauma to the ascending aorta. This therapeutic approach was borrowed from turkey husbandry. Certain strains of turkeys have a high frequency of sudden death due to aortic rupture. It was found in the 1950's that adding reserpine to the turkey food reduced the economic loss. The benefit was thought to be the result of antihypertensive effects of the drug. However, benefit was shown to occur without much reduction in blood pressure, and effect on dP/dT was concluded to be the mechanism. Propranolol was later substituted for reserpine. We believe that, when in the course of annual review patients with the Marfan syndrome are found to have aortic regurgitation, propranolol therapy is indicated. In our series, which now totals about 30 patients, some have been started on propranolol on the basis of dilatation of the aorta demonstrated by echogram or roentgenogram without aortic regurgitation. We attempt to keep the pulse rate in the 60's. The necessary dosage of propranolol is variable, but usually not more than 160 mg. a day. It would appear that the natural history of the progressive aortic dilatation with intercurrent dissection is being altered favorably by the regimen.

In young girls with the Marfan syndrome, puberty has been artificially induced with estrogen (estinyl estradiol) given daily and added progesterone on 4 days at the beginning of each month. The rationale is to prevent excessive growth and also to carry the girl through the period of maximal risk for scoliosis. As a generalization we feel that therapy should be started before age 10; age 4½ years is the youngest patient we have initiated on this program. Questions have been raised regarding the possibility that the hormone therapy increases the risk of aortic rupture, since dissection is seen with greater frequency in pregnant women. In females under the age of 40 years with dissection, half are pregnant or only recently delivered at the time of dissection. Experimental work in rabbits indicates that oral contraceptive agents may have a deleterious effect on the aorta quite separate from their effect on the clotting mechanism. Against the view that the therapy is unreasonably risky is the essentially physiologic dosage used.

*The Ehlers-Danlos syndrome* has turned out to be a highly heterogenous category, characterized by changes in the joints and in the skin. Indeed, at least seven forms are now identifiable, and this clearly does not exhaust the heterogeneity. The joints are hypermobile and the skin is excessively stretchable, fragile, and bruisable.

We now know that rupture of great vessels occurs in at least two of the seven delineated forms of the Ehlers-Danlos syndrome. In type IV Ehlers-Danlos syndrome, otherwise known as the arterial, ecchymotic, or Sack-Barabas type, my colleagues and I (3) have recently shown a thalassemia-like defect in synthesis of type III, or vascular, collagen. In type IV Ehlers-Danlos syndrome, rupture of large arteries is usually not accompanied or preceded by medial dissection but rather is a through-and-through rupture. Furthermore, the rupture involves more frequently the large branches of the aorta such as the innominate or iliac than the aorta itself. True, dissection may occur in the adventitia.

Type IV Ehlers-Danlos syndrome may be itself heterogenous. Some of the experience of Barabas and Beighton suggests dominant inheritance. On the other hand Pope et al. (3) have evidence for recessive inheritance: both parents of a case they studied showed a partial deficiency in synthesis of type III collagen.

We now know that type VI Ehlers-Danlos syndrome, which is inherited as an autosomal recessive and which has as its basic defect deficiency of lysyl hydroxylase, is accompanied by dissecting aneurysm of the aorta. This form of the Ehlers-Danlos syndrome might appropriately be called the ocular form, because fragility of ocular tissues with the rupture of the globe and/or cornea and detachment of the retina, leading to blindness, is a conspicuous feature. I.B.L. (Johns Hopkins Hospital #983764, Figure 6-16 in Reference 1), the patient with type VI Ehlers-Danlos syndrome in whom our group (2) demonstrated lysine hydroxylase deficiency, died at the age of 52 of dissection of the aorta.

One of the reasons that we suspect that this seven-way classification of the Ehlers-Danlos syndrome does not exhaust the heterogeneity in this category of genetic disease is a patient we have seen with type III dissecting aneurysm of the aorta and floppy mitral valve who has severe loose-jointedness in the fingers and other joints, a positive Gorlin sign, stretchable skin and a few somewhat papyraceous scars, all features suggesting the Ehlers-Danlos syndrome (see Figure 6-23 in *Heritable Disorders of Connective Tissue*, 1972). He does, however, not fit into any of the conventional types. His sister died at the age of 53 years following attempted repair of dissecting aneurysm of the aorta. His mother likewise died of dissecting aneurysm at age 53. The sister and the mother had the same loose-jointedness. At least one child of this man has the articular features. The proband died at the age of 55.

The patient illustrated in Figure 1 likewise strains the classification of both the Marfan syndrome and the Ehlers-Danlos syndrome. Of the two conditions, he resembles more the Marfan syndrome. In his youth joint laxity was more marked than is usual in the Marfan syndrome and the type of ocular lesion and the receding jaw are not typical. The Marfanoid hypermobility syndrome (Type III Marfan syndrome) is a possibility. The natural history of that form is not fully characterized.

*Osteogenesis imperfectas* is characterized by brittle bones, blue sclerae, and deafness. It is a generalized disorder of connective tissue as indicated, for example, by the joint laxity. This condition, like the Marfan syndrome and the Ehlers-Danlos syndrome, is undoubtedly heterogeneous. The different forms do not need to concern us here. In one form of congenital osteogenesis imperfecta, my colleagues and I have demonstrated a defect in the synthesis of type I collagen ("collagen vulgaris") (4).

A considerable number of patients with osteogenesis imperfecta tarda have been observed with the floppy mitral valve syndrome and with aortic regurgitation. We have observed one patient who required replacement of the aortic valve for aortic regurgitation. Aortic aneurysm and dissection of the aorta have apparently not been problems in osteogenesis imperfecta.

Probably heritable disorders of connective tissue with serious aortic involvement remain to be delineated.

Familial dissecting aneurysm has been reported in patients without any stigmata of the Marfan syndrome or the Ehlers-Danlos syndrome. Bixler and Antley (5) has studied one such family with dominant transmission and a change in the iris as the only noncardiovascular abnormality: a velvety ectopia of the pigment epithelium around the margin of the pupil and focal pigmented areas of the iris.

The connective tissue features of experimental lathyrism in animals, which is accompanied by aortic aneurysm and rupture, is now known to result from irreversible inhibition of lysyl oxidase, the "crosslinking enzyme" of collagen and elastin, by beta-amino-propionitrile, the toxic substance in the seed of the sweet pea. Deficiency of this enzyme has been claimed in the X-linked form of the Ehlers-Danlos syndrome (6) and in an X-linked form of cutis laxa (8); although the natural history of both awaits

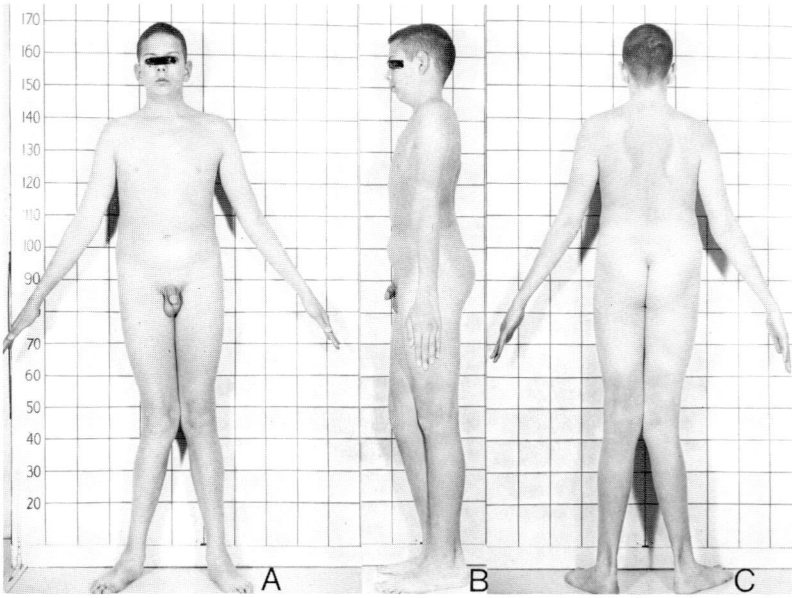


Figure 1. *Marfan-like syndrome* (bilateral retinoschisis, tall stature, arachnodactyly, severe loose-jointedness, genu valgum, scoliosis, spondylolisthesis, and type 3 dissecting aneurysm of aorta).

J.L.D. (JHH 74-95-99), born in 1947, was found, at 18 months of age when he was investigated for strabismus, to have a left "retinal tear." Two operations were performed for correction of the strabismus. Subsequently, "retinal tear" suggesting retinoschisis was discovered in the right eye also. He had only minor refractive error, hyperopic in the left eye and myopic in the right. In 1961 correction of the severe valgus deformity of the knees (A–C) was accomplished by placing of staples in the medial side of the distal femoral metaphyses bilaterally. Hyperextensibility of all joints was marked. Thereafter, two operations for spinal fusion were performed to correct scoliosis. In 1966, a large left inguinal hernia was repaired. Since at least 1971 x-rays have showed severe spondylolisthesis at L-5/S-1.

In 1975 the patient was well and working as a bank manager when he suffered sudden onset of pain in the back. Four days after onset of pain there was radiographic evidence of widening of the mediastinum, and bleeding into the left pleural cavity was confirmed by thoracentesis. Aortogram showed dissection extending from the isthmus into the iliacs. The blood supply of the right kidney was derived from the false channel. With medical therapy the patient's condition was stabilized. He has multiple systolic clicks and echocardiographic changes indicative of "floppy mitral valve." "Pegged lateral incisors" is an independent dominantly inherited trait in this patient, a sister, and their father.

A–C: views in 1961.

full delineation, aortic abnormality has not yet been described. An X-linked mutation in the mouse, referred to by persons who are not mouse geneticists as the "aneurysm-prone mouse" and by mouse geneticists as the "mottled" series, has low lysyl oxidase activity, but the primary defect

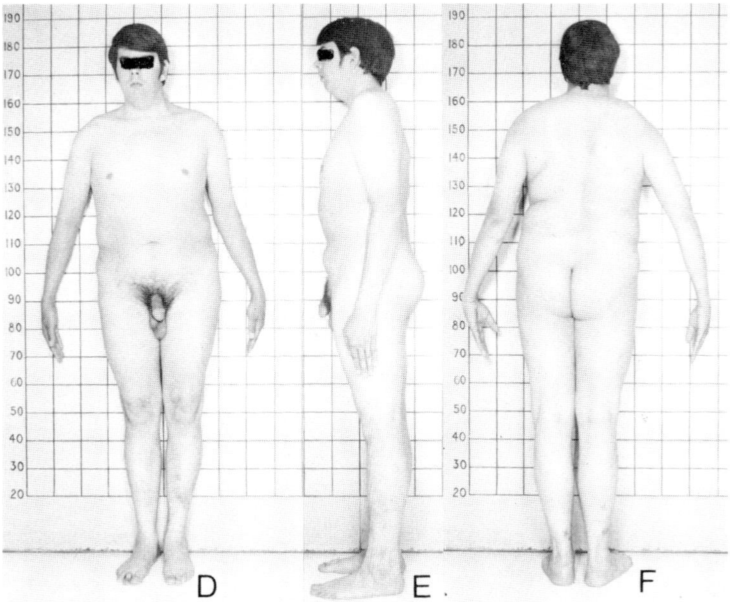

Figure 1D–F. Views in 1971.

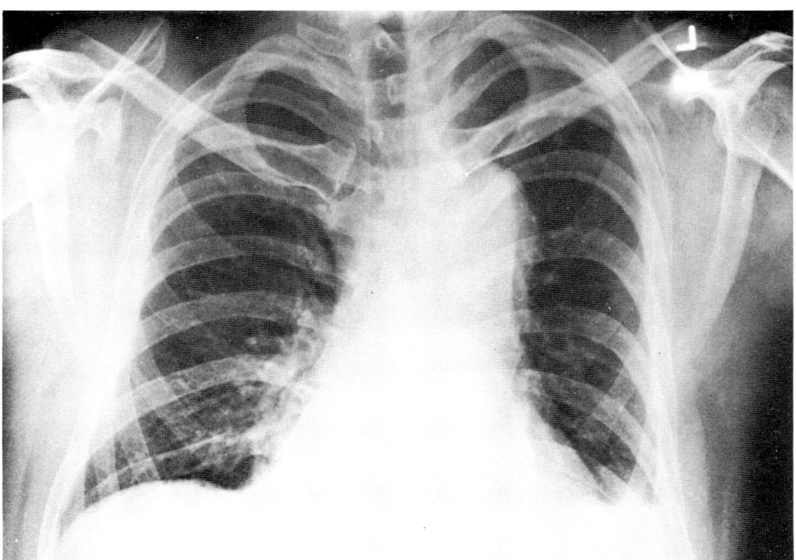

G

Figure 1G. Radiographic view in 1975. X-ray of the chest showing widening of the aortic shadow and left pleural fluid.

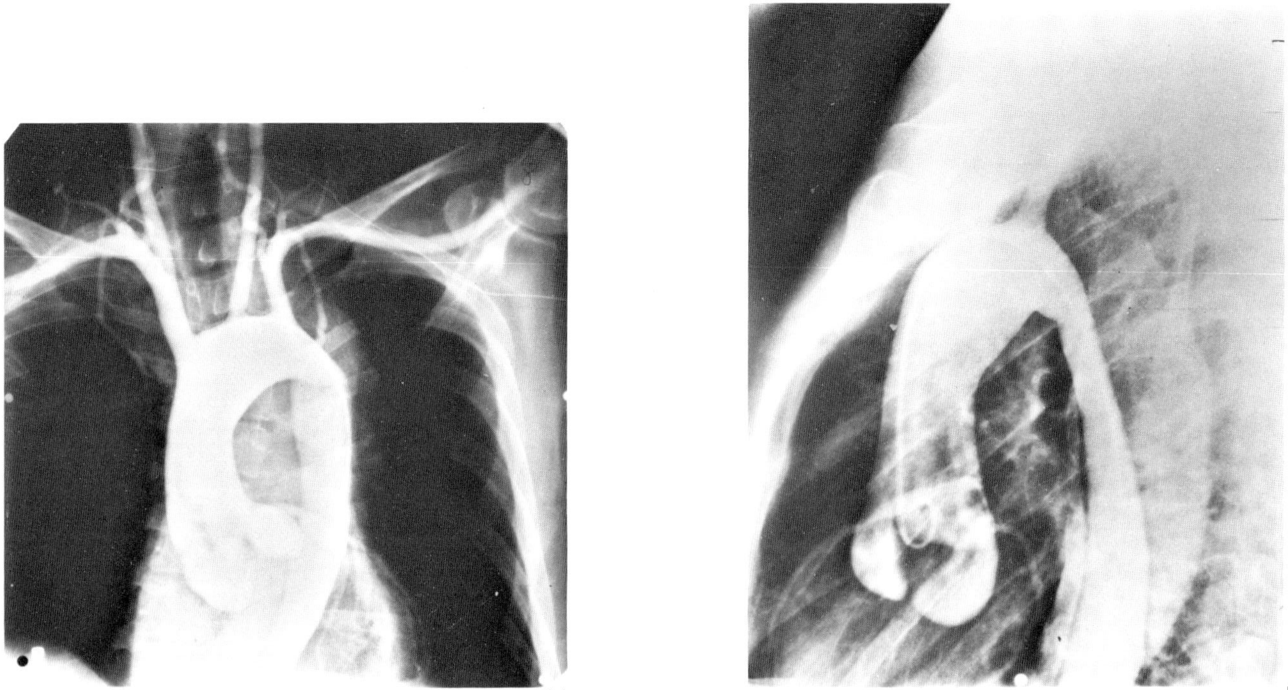

H I

Figure 1H–I. Radiographic views in 1975. Aortogram, in frontal and left anterior oblique projections, showing no dilatation of the first part of the aorta, no aortic regurgitation and no filling of the false channel which lies posteriorly.

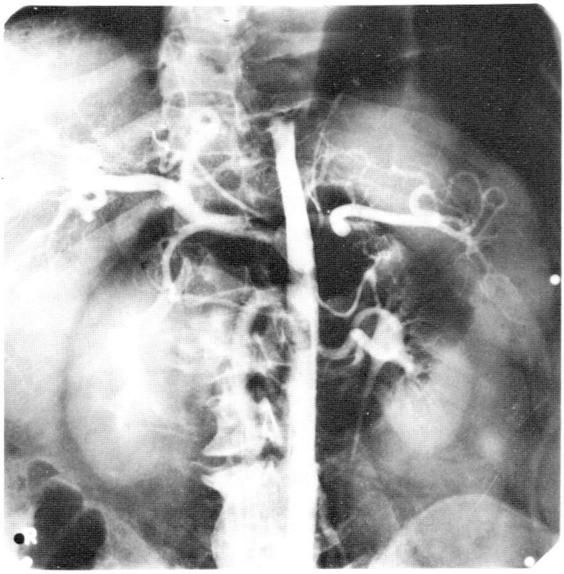

Figure 1J. Radiographic view in 1975. Abdominal aortogram showing that the right kidney is deriving no blood supply from the true channel.

may lie in copper transport across cell membranes. (Lysyl oxidase is a copper-dependent enzyme.)

Cardiovascular surgeons have a unique opportunity to recognize and investigate this group of disorders. The availability of improved techniques for studying the biochemistry of collagen, when combined with heightened interest in and awareness of this category of disease, should result in rapid advances in the next few years.

## REFERENCES

1. McKusick, V. A. 1972. Heritable Disorders of Connective Tissue. Ed. 4, C. V. Mosby Co., St. Louis.
2. Sussman, M. D., Lichtenstein, J. R., Nigra, T. P., et al. 1974. Hydroxylysine-deficient skin collagen in a patient with a form of the Ehlers-Danlos syndrome. J. Bone Joint Surg. 56: 1228–1234.
3. Pope, F. M., Martin, G. R., Lichtenstein, J. R., et al. 1975. Patients with Ehlers-Danlos syndrome type IV lack type III collagen. Proc. Natl. Acad. Sci. USA 72: 1314–1316.
4. Pentinen, R. P., Lichtenstein, J. R., Martin, G. R. et al. 1975. Abnormal collagen metabolism in cultured cells in osteogenesis imperfecta. Proc. Natl. Acad. Sci. USA 72: 586–589.

5. Bixler, D. and Antley, R. M. 1975. Familial dissecting aneurysm. Birth Defects Conference Kansas City, Mo., 4 June. To be published.
6. DiFerrante, N., Leachman, R. D., Angeline, P., Donnelly, P. V., Francis, G., and Almazan, A. 1975. Lysyl oxidase deficiency in Ehlers-Danlos syndrome type V. Connective Tissue Res. 3: 49–53.
7. Byers, P. H., Narayanan, A. S., Bornstein, P., and Hall, J. G. 1975. An X-linked form of cutis laxa due to deficiency of lysyl oxidase, the collagen and elastin crosslinking enzyme. Birth Defects Conference Kansas City, Mo., 4 June. To be published.

# 11 Surgical Therapy of Dissection of the Aorta

N. E. Shumway, M.D., and R. B. Griepp, M.D.

The cause of acute dissection of the aorta is unknown; however, certain associations have been observed. Pregnancy predisposes to a greater incidence as from time to time do such iatrogenic complications as coronary artery endarterectomy utilizing the gas apparatus and aortic or femoral artery cannulation for cardiopulmonary bypass. Marfan's syndrome also may involve intimal tears of the aorta with dissection. Although medial cystic necrosis of the arotic wall is a common finding in dissection, it need not be present in all cases. Arteriosclerosis is often the only pathological finding.

Acute aortic dissection is most commonly observed in middle-aged males. Its incidence has been difficult to determine as so often its symptoms imitate those of myocardial infarction. It is, however, a common entity represented in about five cases/year/million population.

One is suspicious of aortic dissection on the basis of the history and physical examination. The onset of pain is usually sharp and excruciating often indistinguishable from that of myocardial infarction. The presence of an aortic insufficiency murmur, either new or of a changing pattern, is a major physical finding that alerts the clinician, as do changing or paradoxical pulses.

If untreated, aortic dissection is indeed a catastrophic disease. One must distinguish acute aortic dissection from aortic dissecting aneurysm, which is a different entity, a chronic process and one to which the early fenestration operation was applied. Without therapy, only 5% of acute aortic dissections will survive 1 year.

As we have come to understand the prognostic significant of the location of intimal tears in the aorta, we have reclassified acute aortic dissection as 1) an intimal tear of the ascending aorta, 2) a tear in the descending aorta, and 3) a tear which extends into the aortic arch. The majority of lesions are of the first type. A most challenging group of dissections therapeutically are those which present in the ascending or descending aorta and extend beyond into the major arterial branches of the head, into the arch of the aorta.

The approach to therapy consists of immediate institution of antihypertensive medications. Aortography is done in almost all cases although we have operated immediately on a few with obvious new aortic regurgitation murmurs. If the tear involves the ascending aorta, immediate surgery is the treatment of choice. Tears limited to the descending aorta warrant consideration, at least, of medical therapy. There is some disagreement on this issue, and an argument for conservative management can be tolerated.

Surgery aims at preventing rupture of the aorta, the most common cause of death in untreated dissections, and thus is not curative of the underlying disease. In dissections of the ascending aorta, immediate surgery is encouraged, as often the integrity of the aortic valve can be restored, and the need for aortic valve replacement can be circumvented. Resuspension of the aortic valve leaflets is certainly preferable to valve replacement. In the case of dissection accompanied by Marfan's syndrome, valve preservation usually is not possible. The aortic annulus is widely dilated in the Marfan-complicated dissection, and replacement of the ascending aorta and aortic valve is the procedure of choice.

Repair of the ascending or anterior dissection proceeds as follows. Cardiopulmonary bypass is instituted with aortic perfusion through the femoral artery. Retrograde perfusion is maintained while the aorta is cross-clamped, and the heart is cooled by normal saline solution. The aorta is opened, and Teflon bolsters are utilized to resuspend the commissures of the aortic valve. A woven Dacron tube graft is implanted following suture obliteration of the false lumina, both proximal and distal.

In Marfan's syndrome, gross dilatation of the ascending aorta is present, and valve replacement is generally required. We prefer the porcine heterograft valve and woven Dacron for the ascending aortic replacement. In addition, dissection can cause disruption of the right coronary artery from the true lumen. In such a case, a saphenous vein graft can be suspended between the ascending aortic graft and the distal right coronary artery.

Survival in aortic dissection of the ascending aorta treated surgically at the Stanford University Medical Center is 77%. Only 40% survived when medical management alone was utilized. Figure 1 shows the long-term effect of emergency surgery.

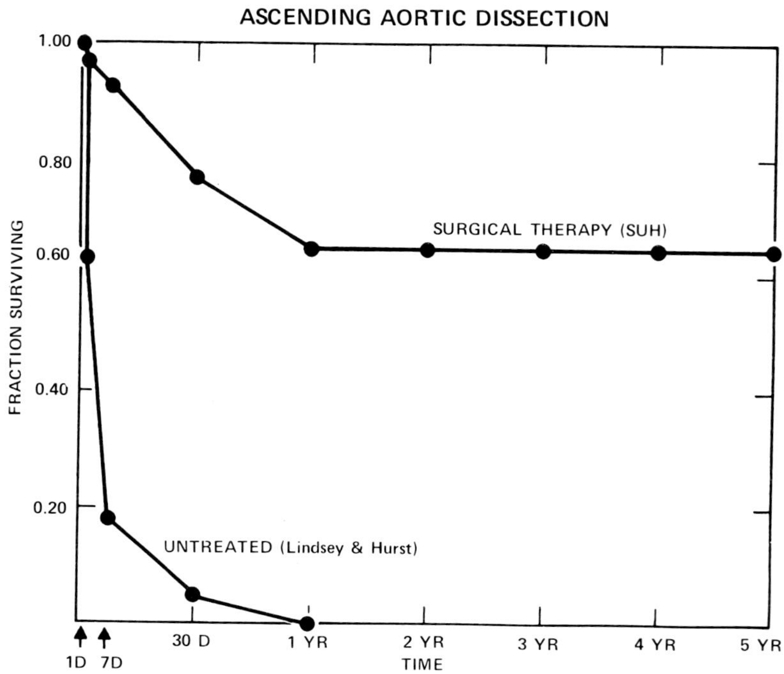


Figure 1. Survival after acute ascending aortic dissection.

Descending aortic dissections carry the additional risk of rupture into the thorax. It is difficult to predict whether or when this will occur, and stable or "healed" dissections of the descending aorta can present with x-ray evidence of tremendous dilatation over a period of years. We prefer, however, to treat most acute posterior dissections of the descending aorta by operation. Partial bypass is employed with femoral artery to femoral vein cannulation. It is imperative in repair of such descending lesions that the true lumen be accurately identified. The false lumen is obliterated by suturing before insertion of the woven Dacron graft.

Factors contributing to the results of therapy include patient age, although we have operated on individuals in the 70's and 80's, and more significantly, the status of the lungs. In surgery of descending dissections requiring 4 to 6 hours, a supine position on the operating table is preferable or a lateral position especially among those with diffuse pulmonary disease. Results at Stanford University Hospital of surgery for posterior dissections are seen in Figure 2.

The final type of dissection is one in which the tear originates in the ascending or descending aorta but extends into the aortic arch. Medical

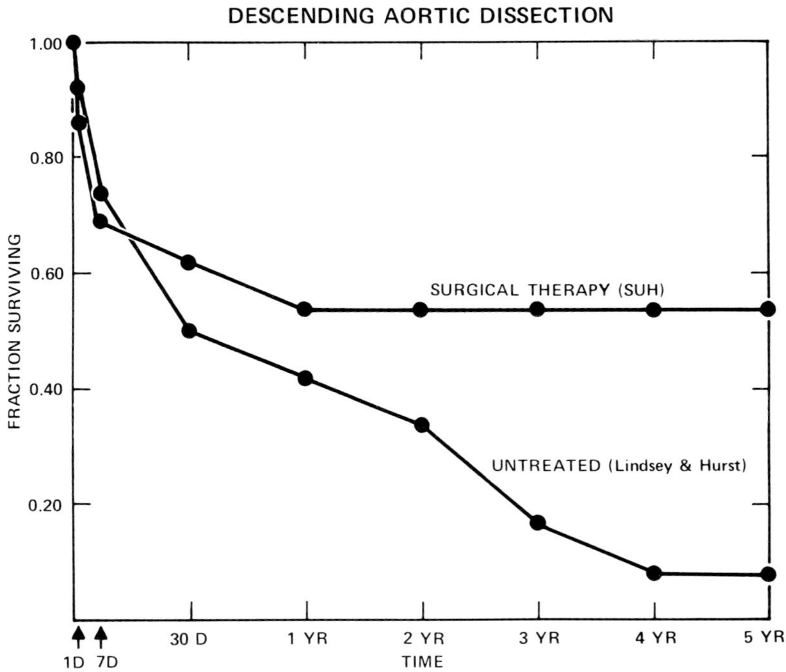


Figure 2. Survival after acute descending aortic dissection.

therapy is uniformly unsuccessful in such cases. The surgical approach to the lesion of ascending-arch tear is as follows. With the patient in a supine position, the femoral vessels are cannulated and cardiopulmonary bypass instituted. The patient temperature is lowered to about 22°C as the ascending aorta is cross-clamped at its most distal portion. The ascending aorta is completely resected, and the aortic valve apparatus resuspended. Replacement of the ascending aorta is accomplished by means of a tubular woven Dacron graft. The proximal anastomosis is carried out at this time. During the procedures described thus far, hypothermic perfusion to the brain has been maintained. At this point, cardiopulmonary bypass is turned off, and under total circulatory arrest lasting up to 30 min. the second phase of the arch reconstruction proceeds. This consists of dissecting free a rim of aortic tissue into which the arch vessels converge. The diseased aortic arch is removed and the distal false lumen of the aorta is obliterated. A second graft is now sutured distally to the descending thoracic aorta, and the aortic button containing the head vessels is sutured into an appropriately tailored opening on the side of this graft. A clamp is then placed across the proximal end of the graft, and cardiopulmonary bypass can be reinstituted while the blood is being warmed. All that remains is to suture the two grafts, one which is now ascending aorta and the other which is arch and first portion of the descending aorta. The combination of circulatory arrest and hypothermia permits complete repair of this lethal condition. The results of arch resection for acute dissection are less satisfactory of course than replacement of either ascending aorta or descending aorta alone. Three cases have been operated upon at Stanford, two of which were long-term survivors. An operative mortality of 33%, nonetheless, compares favorably with the uniform death rate without surgical intervention.

## SUMMARY

Over the past 10 years at Stanford University Hospital a progressively more aggressive surgical approach has been employed for the disease entity appropriately known as acute aortic dissection. The essence of the operation is to remove the site of the intimal tear, to obliterate the false lumina, and to restore aortic continuity by means of a synthetic tubular graft. A convenient and practical classification for acute aortic dissection relates to the site of the intimal tear: 1) ascending aorta, 2) descending aorta, and 3) aortic arch. With the possible exception of the posterior descending group in older patients with diffuse pulmonary disease, immediate surgical intervention is prescribed for all cases of acute aortic dissection.

# 12 Cardiac Anesthesia for Lethal Diseases of the Ascending Aorta

C.-Y. Lin, M.D., and D. W. Benson, M.D.

Moffitt in his review of anesthesia for cardiac surgery noted that essentially every agent and every technique known in anesthesia has been used for cardiac surgery (1). The main principle, regardless of the agent or the technique used, has been light anesthesia. However, we believe that several of the diseases discussed in previous chapters, such as complicated aortic arch disease, main left coronary disease, various types of aortic aneurysms, and transposition of the great vessels, require special attention. Each is an unusually complicated pathophysiological condition of the ascending aorta and we believe that in these circumstances there are some advantages of certain techniques in anesthetic agents over others. This chapter describes the current practices for cardiac anesthesia in these disease situations utilized at The University of Chicago.

## PRESURGICAL MEDICATIONS

Patients with cardiac disease are frequently on several drugs to maintain a functional status in the presence of their disease. A few of these drugs are important because of their interaction with anesthesia and surgery. Perhaps the most important and probably also the most controversial at the present time is propranolol. Viljoen (2) suggested that propranolol should be withheld for 2 weeks prior to coronary surgery because of an experience with five patients receiving propranolol who had unexplained intraoperative cardiac failure. There are several reports of sudden withdrawal of propranolol prior to surgery resulting in severe arrhythmias, angina, and even infarction. At the present time, we have adopted the recommendation of Faulkner (3), who suggests that a withdrawal time of 48 hr. is sufficient for complete recovery from the cardiac effects of propranolol and any possible active metabolites. Coronary bypass surgery under this circumstance had presented no additional hazard. However, in those situations where a patient appears to be truly propranolol dependent, we try not to withdraw the drug completely and recommend that the patient come to surgery under a reduced dose schedule. If the extent of the beta blockade is unknown at the time of anesthesia, a small dose of atropine, such as 0.4 mg. i.v., as well as an isoproterenol test can be tried. If the heart responds by speeding up, in all likelihood the blockade is not severe. For treatment of a severe beta blockade, drugs such as atropine, isoproterenol, or glucagon can be used.

Digitalis is also a controversial drug. We currently feel that it is best to stop any digitalis-type medication 48 hr. prior to surgery. We feel that there are fewer arrhythmias of a serious nature if this routine is followed. Of course, in emergency situations it is not necessary to discontinue the drug.

## PREMEDICATION

The cyanotic patient is said to have an increased sensitivity to sedatives (4). In spite of this, we utilize rather heavy premedication using such drugs and combinations as morphine, scopolamine, and pentobarbital. The usual dose is morphine 0.1 mg. to 0.2 mg./kg., scopolamine 0.01 mg./kg., and pentobarbital 1 mg. to 2 mg./kg. With this, children are usually very calm and will submit to the face mask or will hold it themselves without fight or fear and thus provide a smooth induction. In cyanotic heart disease, a stormy induction can lead to deep cyanosis, which is usually caused by increased airway pressure and a subsequent increase in the right-to-left shunting of blood.

After premedication on the ward, the patients usually receive supplemental oxygen. This is especially true for the cyanotic patient and important during transportation. This is done to ensure that there is no deterioration in oxygenation which might result from an increased anatomical dead space following the use of scopolamine or from a respiratory depression, both in rate and depth, from morphine and pentobarbital. Placement of intravenous needles or catheters is withheld until after induction in children and infants to avoid any unnecessary struggling or anxiety.

For the infant about to undergo deep hypothermia, premedication consists solely of scopolamine 0.1 mg. intramuscularly (i.m.). This is followed by an induction and maintenance with a programmed closed-circuit deep-ether anesthesia sequence and total body surface cooling. In those patients with coronary artery disease, premedication consists of 1 mg./10 kg. body weight of morphine and 1 mg./kg. of pentobarbital plus 0.4 mg. of scopolamine.

## PHYSIOLOGICAL CONSIDERATIONS

Detailed discussion of the principles involved in anesthesia for cardiac surgery are described elsewhere. For the purposes of this discussion, however, it is felt that there are three vital aspects which deserve consideration when anesthetizing the patient with coronary artery disease for open heart surgery or other types of surgery. Needless to say, these points or aspects are just as vital for all other types of heart disease as well. They are:

1. Myocardial oxygen availability
2. Heart rate
3. Hemoglobin content

### Myocardial Oxygen Availability

Recent studies have established the following facts concerning myocardial oxygen demand and supply:

1. Coronary blood flow is influenced by several factors including arterial blood pressure, mainly diastolic pressure; myocardial oxygen consumption and myocardial contractility; blood viscosity and intravascular activating factors. Among these factors, myocardial oxygen consumption is the most important (5, 6).

2. When arterial blood pressure is decreased, coronary blood flow may or may not decrease in a parallel fashion as pressure decreases because of some auto regulation of the coronary system (7, 8).

3. The rate of oxygen extraction is much higher in the myocardium than in other tissues and any increase in myocardial oxygen supply depends chiefly on an increase in coronary blood flow since the oxygen extraction rate is constant; thus, when blood pressure drops during an operative

procedure, the heart is the first organ in which oxygen availability becomes a serious problem (9).

These three factors have contributed to an increase in the use of the intra-aortic ballon before anesthesia in the operating room. The intra-aortic ballon is inserted under local anesthesia. The ballon boosts coronary perfusion by augmentation of the diastolic phase of the arterial pressure and thus reduces the left ventricular work by reducing the peak systolic pressure (10). Introduction of the ballon prior to beginning anesthesia can be carried out smoothly without hypotension. As well as supporting coronary flow during induction and maintenance of anesthesia, the combination of the intra-aortic ballon pumping and extracorporeal circulation has given evidence of superior preservation of the peripheral circulation. This is because perfusion with the pulsatile flow is superior to that with the mean pressure flow of the roller pumps (11, 12).

In the poorly functioning heart following revascularization, the intra-aortic ballon, in general, increases the blood flow through the grafts thereby preventing, to some degree, thrombosis of the grafts. Thus, it is our point of view that we do not hesitate to insert an intra-aortic ballon before revascularization in situations of unstable left main coronary disease with or without shock or in the immediately post revascularization situation where evidence of poor cardiac output exists.

## Heart Rate

Generally, tachycardia reduces the diastolic phase of the cardiac cycle which, in turn, results in an increase of coronary vascular resistance and a decrease in coronary blood flow (13). In the normal heart, an increase in cardiac work resulting from tachycardia increases the myocardial oxygen consumption but initiates a secondary coronary vasodilation and thus maintains the supply of oxygen to the myocardium. In the case of coronary occlusion, however, this balance between supply and demand may not occur and a myocardial oxygen debt may result. Katz and Feinberg (14) have shown that oxygen consumption in the heart is directly related to the product of heart rate and peak systolic pressure. This situation usually applies when the tachycardia is the result of sympathetic overactivity. In the diseased heart, however, these simple relationships may not apply. Thus, tachycardia is something that should be avoided if possible.

At the opposite end of the scale, bradycardia produces a not dissimilar situation. For example, Sandler and Ghista (15) have demonstrated that the myocardial oxygen requirement increases when myocardial wall tension increases with bradycardia since the chambers fill to a greater degree and cardiac output fails to match the control conditions. Thus, if a patient has the complication of a recent atrioventricular block and has coronary artery disease, a temporary transvenous pacemaker is inserted prior to surgery to maintain an adequate heart rate and thus decrease myocardial wall tension.

## Hemoglobin Content

In all forms of heart disease, but especially in patients having coronary artery disease, hemoglobin content of the blood is important. Myocardial oxygen extraction goes on at a much higher rate in the heart than in other organs and stays fairly constant at a level of 70 to 80%, in spite of fluctuations in the arterial oxygen content. Arterial oxygen content, of course, depends on hemoglobin content and its saturation. Oxygen saturation is determined by the arterial oxygen partial pressure available to the blood and the configuration of the hemoglobin dissociation curve. Several investigators have demonstrated that the maximum oxygen delivery to tissue including the myocardium is obtained when hematocrit is between 35 and 40% (16). Thus, in the case of coronary artery disease, one should endeavor to have the hemoglobin content of the blood between 13 and 15 g./100 ml. (35 to 40% hematocrit).

When the hematocrit exceeds 50%, there can be deleterious effects on the coronary circulation. The viscosity of the blood is sharply increased when the hematocrit reaches or exceeds 50%, and there will be a marked increase in resistance to coronary flow, a slowing of the flow, and a decrease in available oxygen. This effect, caused by the high viscosity, becomes more prominent in patients with coronary artery disease because of the obstruction in these vessels. Distal to the narrowing of the coronary arteries there is a marked decrease in the shear rate, and the change in viscosity becomes exaggerated. These changes can be further aggravated by any transient hypotension that might occur during the induction or maintenance of anesthesia and surgery (17).

Thus great care must be taken to ascertain the hemoglobin content of blood and maintain it at a level that allows for optimal oxygen transfer and minimal effects of increased viscosity. This is especially important in the coronary patient who has received vigorous medical management utilizing diuretics to control fluid build-up and the failing heart. These patients may have a sudden increase in viscosity of the blood resulting from the hemoconcentration, and this may invoke new obstructions distal to narrowing in the coronary arteries.

## INDUCTION AND MAINTENANCE OF ANESTHESIA

Maintenance of a stable circulatory status from the induction of anesthesia to the beginning of extracorporeal circulation is very important in the anesthetizing of critical cardiac cases for open heart surgery. All of the anesthetic sequences utilized possess in varying degrees the capability of myocardial depression and/or peripheral vascular dilatation. This includes premedication since, although a tranquil state is desirable for induction of anesthesia, it must not be obtained at the expense of undue respiratory or cardiovascular depression. Although in our practice we choose various agents according to the physical status of the patients, we also tend to choose the agents and the techniques according to the disease entity because the pathophysiology may cause a different cardiopulmonary status from disease to disease.

For the following conditions, we generally choose the anesthesia as listed unless it is contraindicated by yet another factor:

1. Coronary artery disease
   a. Morphine, muscle relaxant, nitrous oxide and oxygen
   b. Innovar, muscle relaxant, nitrous oxide and oxygen
2. Acute aortic dissections
   a. Halothane, muscle relaxant, oxygen (with or without nitrous oxide and narcotics)
3. Transposition of great vessels
   a. For shunt operation
      1. Halothane, muscle relaxants, and oxygen
      2. Ketamine, muscle relaxants, and oxygen
4. For total correction with deep hypothermia
   a. Diethyl ether, oxygen, closed circuit

## ANESTHESIA WITH MORPHINE AS THE MAIN AGENT

All patients are preoxygenated. Induction is begun with small doses of morphine, usually 0.4 mg. to 1 mg./kg. body weight, given at the rate of 5 mg./min. The blood pressure, electrocardiogram, and mental status are monitored continuously. Very early in our experience with morphine anesthesia, we noted two cases of unusual sensitivity to morphine manifested by prolonged neurological depression which had to be reversed by very large doses of naloxone. Thus, since that time we have used small doses of morphine and have stopped the induction when the patient responds to command by scarcely opening his eyelids. This dose rarely exceeds 1 mg./kg. body weight.

When the patient is stable, 50 to 100 mg. of thiopental is given intravenously followed by 1 mg./kg. of succinylcholine to facilitate intubation. Immediately after intubation, a nondepolarizing muscle relaxant, pancuronium, is given in the dose of 0.5 mg./kg., unless the basic pulse rate in adults exceeds 100/min. When the heart rate is greater than 100/min., *d*-tubocurare is sometimes used for neuromuscular paralysis, especially in reasonably healthy candidates. Anesthesia maintenance is then continued with nitrous oxide and oxygen at flows of 3 L and 2 L/min., respectively, for approximately 15 min. The semiclosed system is then changed to a closed circuit with low flows, and oxygen concentration of 40% is maintained. This is done to preserve the humidity in the system for the airway. The lungs are ventilated mechanically at a rate of 12/min., with tidal volumes of 10 to 15 cc./kg.

The initial morphine is supplemented with a 10-mg. dose given just before the skin incision. If marked hypertension develops following the surgical incision, suggesting excessive sympathetic activity that is not suppressible with further administration of morphine, halothane in concentrations generally less than 1% is added to the breathing circuit. This type of response is quite often seen in the healthier group of patients and it is felt that by maintaining the systolic pressure at rate of 120 to 140 mm. Hg, the work load on the heart is considerably less.

There have been several reports concerning the antidiuretic hormone-stimulating effect of morphine (18, 19). Our results would indicate that there is no statistically significant difference between such agents as innovar, morphine, and halothane in this respect (20). Our own studies indicate that the ratio of urine output to the amount of infusion is the same for all of them.

## INNOVAR

Innovar is administered at the rate of 1 cc./3 min., with a total dose of approximately 2 to 4 cc. Quite often following the administration of innovar, blood pressure will drop dramatically, especially in chronic coronary disease patients. This is probably related to the alpha-blocking properties of droperidol, which overcome the sympathetic overactivity often seen in chronic heart failure. Usually volume replacement corrects this situation well. Too rapid injection of innovar is usually the cause of such an effect. Intubation follows after 50 to 100 mg. of thiopental intravenous and 1 mg./kg. of succinylcholine.

After the innovar induction, only rarely is more than 100 mg. of thiopental required to abolish the lash reflex. Obviously, the thiopental should be given slowly and one should wait longer than normally to evaluate the dose response because of the slow circulation time. Following intubation, a nondepolarizing neuromuscular blocking agent is added and fentanyl is administered as needed. Again, ventilation is maintained automatically with a volume of 10 to 15 cc./kg. at the rate of 12/min. Nitrous oxide is used for maintenance at a concentration of 60%.

## HALOTHANE

Light halothane anesthesia coupled with relaxants is still an important choice for a variety of situations. This is true mainly because it provides an easy control over blood pressure and, especially in children, gives a rapid, smooth induction (21). Thus, in most pediatric cardiac anesthesia, halothane is the agent of choice. In most of the surgery on aortic-arch aneurysms, halothane is also the preferred agent. This is the case because most of the patients with such disease have severe hypertension and the blood pressure must be maintained within reasonable limits. Except for aneurysms involving the transverse arch, the techniques are straightforward and essentially the same as with other agents. The transverse arch presents considerable anatomical variations and the anesthetic technique must be flexible to adjust for these varying circumstances, such as regional cooling, selective perfusion, and the like. A detailed discussion of the anesthesia technique is described by Paulissian and Anagnostopoulos (22).

## ANESTHESIA FOR DEEP HYPOTHERMIA

Since 1971, we have used a closed circuit technique for the administration of diethyl ether for infants undergoing cardiac surgery in deep hypothermia and total cardiac arrest (23). Briefly, this technique consists of calculating a total dose of diethyl ether utilizing Lowe's formula, which will give a concentration in the blood of 2 times the minimum alveolar concentration within 30 to 60 min (24). The ether is injected into the circuit with a syringe pump programmed to inject rapidly at first, when uptake is at its highest, and then to taper off the rate of injection with time. The concentration of ether is monitored in the expiratory limb of the anesthesia circuit with a concentration monitor known as a Narcotest, and the concentration is kept at approximately a 5% level. At 40 min., the 5% respiratory concentration will accurately be reflected by the concentration of ether in the blood as measured by a gas chromatograph.

To use this technique, the patients are intubated prior to commencing the ether anesthesia. Neonates are intubated while awake after oxygenation and infants are intubated following a 2 mg./kg. dose of succinylcholine administered intramuscularly. After intubation the patients are attached to the anesthesia circuit, which is then closed, and a flow of oxygen just slightly more than the metabolic needs of the patient is admitted via a needle valve. The ventilation is assisted by hand, and the diethyl ether is administered by the syringe pump at a pre-programmed rate.

When the patient is well anesthetized, two intravenous routes are started and an arterial line is established. A Foley catheter is inserted. Two temperature probes, one in the rectum and one in the esophagus, are also inserted. The sacrum of the infant is padded with several thicknesses of 4 X 4 gauze to minimize the effects of the cooling environment on the temperature probe in the rectum. The amount of tissue between the outside environment and the rectal mucosa in the infant is minimal and the temperature will read lower than what the core temperature actually is.

Surface cooling is achieved by placing the patient on a platform that can be lowered directly into ice water. The posterior part of the body is lowered into the water and several plastic bags of ice are placed on the anterior surface of the body. The ice bags are removed at a temperature of 25°C, and the skin is prepared, draped, and the incision is made while the posterior parts of the body are still in contact with the ice water. The temperature will continue to drop, but the platform should be raised at a point 2 to 3° above the final expected temperature to allow for drift.

During cooling the solubility of the anesthetic agent increases. The rate of ether administration, therefore, must be adjusted accordingly. For example, at 30°C, the narcotest should read at the 3% level and at 20°C at the 2% level. This would coincide with a level of 5% at normal body temperature.

The following measures are carried out during the surface cooling to protect from hemoconcentration and possible renal damage:

1. 2 ml./kg. of lactated Ringers solution administered intravenously for every degree drop of rectal temperature from 35 to 25°C.
2. Lasix, 5 mg. just before cooling and another 5 mg. at 30°C.
3. Manitol, 1.5 g. at 30 and 25°C.

We have utilized this technique in more than 100 neonates and infants of less than 8 kg. body weight for the correction of complicated cardiac anomalies. We have never encountered ventricular fibrillation or cardiac arrest. The patients are generally very hemodynamically stable and the heart has stayed in sinus rhythm throughout the cooling phase. In contrast to other anesthesia techniques, the lack of irritability during handling of the heart prior to the intracardiac surgery is remarkable. When the desired temperature has been achieved, total cardiac arrest is obtained after occlusion of the venae cavae and ascending aorta by injecting several milliliters of Young's solution into the root of the aorta proximal to the aortic occlusion clamp. Safe total cardiopulmonary arrest can be achieved at a core temperature of approximately 20°C for approximately 1 hr.

Following completion of the intracardiac corrective surgery, rewarming is achieved by both core and surface warming. The heat exchanger in the pump is used for core warming and the temperature difference between the water and the blood is maintained at no greater than 10°C to avoid possible liberation of gas bubbles in the blood. No more ether is administered to the patient after cardiac arrest.

## MANAGEMENT DURING PERFUSION

### Priming

We routinely use a non-blood prime for the extracorporeal pump. A balanced electrolyte solution in the amount recommended for the oxygenator being used is put into the pump initially. We may add blood to maintain a hemoglobin content of not less than 8 g.% and will add blood ahead of time if the patient is known to be anemic to such a degree that the diluted blood will have a hemoglobin of less than 8 g.%.

### Heparinization

Just before cannulation, 3 mg./kg. of a beef lung preparation of heparin are administered into the circulation. Half of this initial dose of heparin is administered every hour thereafter for the duration of the pumping period. As experience accumulates, however, we should be able to monitor heparin levels through the activated clotting time measurement.

### Perfusion Flow Rate and Pressures

In general, we endeavor to pump at a rate of 2.2 to 2.5 L/M$^2$ of body surface area. In cyanotic patients, we add another 10 to 20% to compensate for bronchial flow. Arterial cannula selection is a critical factor and we utilize cannulae that will allow us to maintain a flow as suggested above, but with a line pressure from the pump, of less than 200 mm. Hg. The lower the line pressure that can be maintained, the less likelihood of a cavitation effect and shear stress on the red cell in the cannula during perfusion and thus the less likelihood of damage to the red cells.

### Monitoring during Bypass

During perfusion, we monitor the following parameters:
1. Arterial pressure
2. Central venous pressure
3. Line pressure
4. Body temperature and blood temperature
5. Flow rate
6. Urine output
7. Frequent blood gases

## TERMINATION OF CARDIOPULMONARY BYPASS

Before completion of cardiopulmonary bypass, the flow is gradually reduced, carefully following the blood pressure and observing the cardiac action. During this time or shortly before, 500 mg. of calcium chloride in the adult, or 300 mg. in the young child, is put into the pump and given approximately 5 min. to equilibrate. The vital signs, such as the central venous pressure, blood pressure, pupils, temperature, and so on, are checked and their condition noted. Blood is prepared for transfusion. The lungs are hyperinflated several times.

The pump is brought to a standstill and adequate transfusion from the pump is given. Pharmacological support is rarely used after termination of cardiopulmonary bypass. However, we do feel free to use pharmacological support if there is any doubt of circulatory stability. Relieving intense vasoconstriction during the pumping procedure with the appropriate anesthesia or with mild alpha blockers is an important factor in reducing the use of pharmacological support in the post-perfusion period. If a high peripheral resistance is present at this time, a weak myocardium that may have been insulted with hypoxia during the operative procedure may not have the power to overcome such resistance.

If a vasoactive drug is essential, the drug of choice at the present time is dopamine. It is given by a continuous intravenous infusion at a rate of 10 μg./kg./min. Recent experimental work has demonstrated that, in induced myocardial infarctions, the use of peripheral constrictors and beta adrenergic blockade decreased the size of the infarction. On the other hand, catecholamines with their inotropic action caused an extension of the infarction. Our clinical experience also supports the use of a peripheral constrictor, rather than isoproternol in cardiogenic shock (25, 26). The heparin that was administered for perfusion is neutralized with protamine in a ratio of 1.5–2 to 1 mg./mg. of the initial dose of heparin. The protamine is injected slowly over a period of approximately 10 min. to minimize the possibility of hypotension and direct myocardial depression and increased pulmonary vascular resistance. We frequently administer 500 mg. to 1 g. of calcium chloride just prior to the protamine administration to avoid any direct myocardial depression from the protamine.

## MANAGEMENT AFTER CARDIOPULMONARY BYPASS

In the immediate post-perfusion period, the patients rarely require anesthesia of any greater potency than 50% nitrous oxide. Blood gases are taken while the patient is ventilated on 100% oxygen to determine the presence of any shunting that might require an elevated oxygen concentration during the immediate postoperative period. Also, if there is any deviation from normal in the acid base status, it is corrected at this time generally with sodium bicarbonate. The milliequivalent dose of sodium bicarbonate to be given is calculated by the formula, the base deficit in milliequivalents times the body weight in kilograms divided by six.

Blood replacement is guided by the circulatory response of the patient. The venous pressure is probably the greatest help in following the tranfusion response, and it also contributes to an understanding of the heart function and efficiency. A judgment is made on the basis of the arterial pressure and the venous pressure on whether to give blood transfusion. Except for valvular disease, a left atrial pressure line is seldom inserted for following postoperative blood transfusion. In these instances, however, it is felt that the left atrial pressure is extremely important when replacing blood.

In aortic aneurysm surgery, an inhalation anesthetic such as halothane is frequently used to control high blood pressure, which is often seen following bypass. These patients, for reasons that are unclear, frequently have vasoconstriction and the use of vasoconstrictors to support blood pressure is truly contraindicated in these patients.

Routinely, patients who have undergone cardiopulmonary bypass in cardiac surgery are ventilated at least over night with a volume-limited ventilator to reduce the work cost of breathing and to make it possible to assess the postoperative circulatory status under optimal respiratory conditions. A tidal volume of 10 to 15 cc./kg. body weight with a rate of 12/min. is the initial setting. Oxygen in a concentration of 40% is administered at the beginning and after the measurement of blood gases is adjusted up or down to maintain a $pO_2$ of at least 60 mm. Hg. It is necessary to maintain a reasonable lung volume so that if the $pCO_2$ is lower than 35 mm. Hg., mechanical dead space is added between the ventilator and the endotracheal tube.

The size of the dead space necessary is derived by first calculating the minute alveolar ventilation from the following relationship:

$$\frac{\text{arterial } pCO_2}{\text{barometric pressure} - \text{water vapor pressure}} = \frac{CO_2 \text{ production}}{(\text{tidal volume} - \text{physiological dead space}) \times \text{resp. rate}}$$

thus:

$$\text{physiological dead space} = \text{tidal vol.} - \frac{CO_2 \text{ production} \times (\text{barometric pressure} - \text{water vapor pressure})}{\text{arterial } pCO_2 \times \text{respiratory rate}}$$

Then the mechanical dead space needed to achieve 40 mm. arterial $pCO_2$ is:

$$\text{mechanical dead space} = \frac{(40 - \text{arterial } pCO_2)(\text{tidal volume} - \text{physiological dead space})}{40}$$

To simplify these calculations, we assume a $CO_2$ production in the adult of 3 cc./kg./min. and water vapor pressure of 42 mm. Hg.

## MONITORING

In the adult patient, a central venous line is passed through the antecubital vein. If this is impossible, after the patient is anesthetized, a catheter is inserted into the external jugular vein for measuring central venous pressure. A 20-gauge plastic needle is passed percutaneously into the radial artery for measuring arterial pressure and blood gases. Other monitors are the electrocardiogram, rectal temperature, uninary output, blood gases, and electrolytes. In some few cases, the left atrial pressure is monitored, but generally this is in the postoperative period. The electroencephalogram and cardiac output are also occasionally monitored. The latter is done by the thermodilution technique. During extracorporeal circulation, both the mixed venous and arterial blood gases are monitored at 15- to 30-min. intervals to determine the performance of the oxygenator and also to get an indication of the adequacy of perfusion.

## REFERENCES


1. Moffitt, E. A., Tarhan, S., and Lundborg, R. O. 1968. Anesthesia for cardiac surgery. Anesthesiology 29: 1181.
2. Viljoen, J. F., Estafanous, F., and Kellner, G. A. 1972. Propranolol and cardiac surgery. J. Thorac. Cardiovasc. Surg. 64: 826.
3. Faulkner, S. L., Hopkins, J. T., Boerth, R. C., Young, J. L., Jr., Jellett, L. B., Nies, A. S., Bender, H. W., and Shand, D. G. 1973. Time required for complete recovery from chronic propranolol therapy. New Engl. J. Med. 289: 607.
4. Lowenstein, E., Walker, H. L., and Zarloff, L. I. 1965. The effect of a standard cyanotic circulatory lesion on the induction dose of mehhoxital in the dog. Anesthesiology 26: 254.
5. Feinberg, H., and Katz, L. N. 1958. Effect of cathecholamines L-epinephrine and l-norepinephorine on coronary blood flow and oxygen metabolism of the myocardium. Am. J. Physiol. 193: 151.
6. Allela, A., Williams, F. L., Bolene-Williams, C., and Katz, L. N. 1955. Interrelation between cardiac oxygen consumption and coronary blood flow. Am. J. Physiol. 183: 570.
7. Ross, J., Jr., Mosher, P. W., and Shaw, R. F. 1961. Autoregulation of coronary blood flow circulation. 24: 1025.
8. Berne, R. M. 1964. Regulation of coronary blood flow. Physiol. Rev. 44: 1.
9. Nakamura, Y., Tkahashi, M., Takei, F., Matsumura, N., Scholkens, B., and Sasamoto, H. The change in coronary vascular resistance during acute induced hypoxia—with special reference to coronary vascular reserve. Cardologia 54: 91.
10. Galysh, F. T., Garyin, P. J., Lin, C. Y., and Patel, A. S. 1969. Study of the physiological effects of circulatory assist devices. Annual Technical Progress Report No. BX-14-25-69A.
11. Pappas, G., Winter, S. D., Kopriva, C. J., and Steele, P. P. 1975. Improvement of myocardial and other vital organ functions and metabolism with a simple method of pulsatile flow (I.A.B.P.) during clinical cardiopulmonary bypass. Surgery 77: 34.
12. Anagnostopoulos, C. E., Lin, C. Y., Lamberti, J. J., Replogle, R. L., and Skinner, D. B. 1975. Expanding indications for intra-aortic balloon diastolic augmentation. J. Eur. Soc. Surg. Res. April, 1975.
13. McGregor-Palmer, W. H. 1963. Mechanism of angina pectoris. *In* Likoff, W. and Moyer, J. H. (Eds.). Coronary Heart Disease, p. 178. Grune and Stratton, New York.
14. Katz, L. N., and Feinberg, H. 1958. Relation of cardiac effort to myocardial $O_2$ consumption and coronary flow. Circ. Res. 6: 656.
15. Sandler, H., and Ghista, D. N. 1969. Mechanical and dynamic implications of dimensional measurements of the left ventricle. Fed. Proc. 28: 1349.
16. Richardson, T. Q., and Guyton, A. C. 1959. Effects of polycythemia and anemia on cardiac output and other circulatory factors. Am. J. Physiol. 197: 1167.
17. Dintenfass, L. 1967. Rheology of blood in cardiovascular disease. Bibl. Anat. 9: 525.

18. Papper, S., and Papper, E. M. 1964. The effects of pre-anesthetic anesthetic and postoperative drugs on renal function. Clin. Pharmacol. Ther. 5: 205.
19. Stanley, T. H., Gray, N. H., Stanford, W., and Armstrong, R. 1973. The effect of high-dose morphine on fluid and blood requirements in open heart operation. Anesthesiology 38: 536.
20. Lin, C. Y., Paulissian, R., and Mostert, J. W. Comparative study on morphine, innovar and haolthane anesthesia on fluid requirement in open heart surgery. (Unpublished data.)
21. Strong, M. J., Keat, A. S., and Cooley, D. A. 1966. Anesthesia for cardiovascular surgery in infancy. Anesthesiology 27: 257.
22. Paulissian, R. and Anagnostopoulos, C. E. 1975. Anesthesia for acute aortic dissection. *In* Anagnostopoulos, C. E. (Ed.). Acute Aortic Dissections, p. 142. University Park Press, Batimore.
23. Lin, C. Y., Paulissian, R., and Lowe, H. (Unpublished data.)
24. Lowe, H. 1972. Dose-regulated penthrane anesthesia. Abbott Lab., p. 58.
25. Maroko, P. R., Kjekshus, J. K., and Sobel, B. E. 1971. Factors influencing infarct size following experimental coronary artery occlusion. Circulation 63: 67.
26. Mueller, H., Ayres, S. M., and Gregory, J. J. 1970. Hemodynamics, coronary blood flow and myocardial metabolism in coronary shock response to l-novepinepherine and isoproterenol. J. Clin. Invest. 49: 1885.

# 13
# Panel on Acute Aortic Dissection

**Moderator**
D. A. Cooley, M.D.
**Panel Members**
V. A. McKusick, M.D., N. E. Shumway, M.D.,
and C. E. Anagnostopoulos, M.D.

**Dr. Cooley**: I am certain that you have all enjoyed hearing from these experts on the subject of acute aortic dissection. I would like to open this session by asking Dr. McKusick whether any successful surgical procedures have been accomplished in patients with the Ehlos-Danler's syndrome. It continues to be the surgeon's nemesis and my own experience has been rather disastrous in operating on these patients since the vessels are particularly friable, to a greater extent than seen even in Marfan's syndrome.

**Dr. McKusick**: I agree that the quality of the vessels seen in this disorder make surgical attempts at repair quite difficult. These patients seem to profit from medical therapy.

**Dr. Cooley**: I am interested in the indications for medical therapy mentioned by Dr. Anagnostopoulos. I would tend to take issue with him on this point. I believe the only indications for such therapy are refusal for surgery by the patient or the unavailability of a surgical team at the time of the castastrophe. On the basis of odds alone, the therapy for dissection should be surgical. There may be a question of timing, whether the operation should be done now or in the morning, but the presence of dissection is the indication for early surgical intervention. There is nothing more frustrating to the surgeon than rupture of the aorta in a patient being treated medically who presented hours earlier with the classic findings of dissection.

I was interested in Dr. Shumway's slide review of current surgical management of dissection. I noted particularly that a pocket of dissected aorta is left behind, both proximally and distally. This is very worrisome to the surgeons and I wonder if he is concerned about increase in the size of the distal pocket. We use a collar graft around the outer vessel to prevent this occurrence. Dr. Shumway, do you believe in reinforcement of the remaining aortic segments during repair?

**Dr. Shumway**: I believe this is useful and especially in Marfan's syndrome where dissection is usually limited to the ascending aorta alone. But in those cases where re-entry of the dissection has occurred in the diaphragmatic area or just below, the best we can hope for is that the false lumen will clot. Heading off the disastrous sequelae of acute dissection by prompt surgical therapy to prevent early death is still the most that we can do.

**Dr. Cooley**: One of the major problems that faces the cardiovascular surgeon is that of maintaining cerebral viability while the circulation is interrupted. In high risk patients, it has been my experience that cooling to 12 or 16°C does not necessarily prevent decerebrate rigidity postoperatively. I am personally somewhat reluctant to accept a period of ischemia of 30 min. with the patient at 20°C. Certain alternatives might, therefore, be useful. I believe the transverse arch is a relatively safe area as far as rupture is concerned, and perhaps the area of the major visceral vessels of the abdominal area as well. One might consider, even though it appears to be a retrograde step, wrapping of the transverse arch and then resection of the ascending or descending aorta. Dr. Shumway, will you comment?

**Dr. Shumway**: We all can comment about patients who do not wake up following surgery. This can be related to many factors other than the period of ischemia during circulatory arrest. For example, we operated on a man who had an absent right carotid pulse but was conscious on admission to the hospital. He had an ascending aortic tear and the usual operation for repair was accomplished with ease and dispatch. However, after surgery he became decerebrate. We believe that reactive hyperemia probably occurred in the brain following re-establishment of blood flow to the right carotid artery, and thus the brain became edematous with total loss of cerebral function. So the fact that a patient does not awaken postoperatively may be entirely unrelated to cooling and its effect on the brain.

**Dr. Anagnostopoulos:** I would like to comment further on wrapping of the aortic arch in dissection. We recently treated a 10-year-old child with Marfan's syndrome in whom rupture of the arch had occurred. Following femorofemoral bypass we dissected the entire ascending arch and descending aorta via a lateral thoracotomy since there was prominent scoliosis. There was aortic insufficiency and it was unclear whether we should replace the arch and valve. Instead, we wrapped the arch to prevent rupture and exsanguination. The wrapping was carried far down proximally to eliminate aortic insufficiency. The patient is alive 6 months later, and this points to the usefulness of aortic wrapping in select cases.

**Dr. Cooley:** Dr. McKusick, in addition to medical therapy, is there a place for more radical treatment in those patients with Marfan's in whom the clear cut indications for surgical therapy have not yet developed?

**Dr. McKusick:** The idea of wrapping the aorta before the occurrence of an aneurysm is certainly an intriguing idea but at this stage I would probably pass the wrapping stage. However, perhaps this should be reconsidered.

**Dr. Cooley:** Several bizarre forms of therapy have been considered and applied in acute aortic dissection. It is still the surgeon's dilemma. We operated on two patients with dissection of the ascending aorta who posed a very special problem. After bypass was instituted, the ascending aorta was opened but it appeared to consist only of adventitia; there was no internal lumen. So we turned the pump off and reached down inside the aortic arch and the descending aorta and pulled a sleeve of dissected intima back into position and proceeded with the repair in the usual manner. So dissections can take on many forms. We treated one patient whom we made into a surgical career. A courageous woman came to us 10 years ago when she was 36 years old with an acute dissection of her ascending aorta which we repaired. She returned with an abdominal aneurysm because the lower end of her dissection process had enlarged and so we resected her abdominal aorta. Several years later she came back with an expanding lesion in the descending thoracic aorta and we replaced her descending aorta. About a year ago she presented again with aortic regurgitation and a huge aneurysm proximal to our previous anastomosis. We replaced the aortic annulus, reimplanted both coronary arteries and replaced the aortic valve. The lesson is simply that you must plug up all leaks as they occur.

**Question from the floor:** Was this patient hypertensive?

**Dr. Cooley**: No, she was normotensive throughout her hospital course. I am sure that antihypertensive therapy is important in the medical management of this disorder, but I am not as certain of long-term propranolol. Decreasing myocardial contractility seems a bit of a paradox at times. Dr. McKusick, will you comment?

**Dr. McKusick**: Obviously one should not use digitalis in combination with propranolol as these would work against each other. Long-term propranolol therapy does seem to be effective and several patients with even aortic insufficiency have been treated for up to 10 years with this agent.

**Dr. Cooley**: Weakening the muscle therapeutically is nothing new. I remember in the treatment of claudication those who severed the Achilles tendon and found that if you could not contract your calf muscles you would not claudicate when you walked!

I would like to leave you with this thought in closing. Acute aortic dissection can take on many forms and with our limited knowledge we must attempt to apply the proper therapy to the particular patient. Thank you.

# Index

Anatomy, left main coronary artery, 2
Anesthesia, cardiac
  for deep hypothermia, 136–138
  halothane, 136
  heart rate, 132–133
  hemoglobin content, 133
  induction and maintenance, 134
  Innovar, 135–136
  for lethal diseases of ascending aorta, 129–143
  management during perfusion, 138–139
  with morphine as main agent, 134–135
  myocardial oxygen availability, 131–132
  physiological considerations, 131–133
  premedication, 130–131
  pre-infarction, in left main coronary artery disease, 18–26
    angiography, 21–22
    clinical material, 19
    definitions, 18
    hemodynamic data, 20
    results of treatment, 23–25
    treatment, 22–23
  unstable, 37–48
    clinical course and management, 39–40
    clinical spectrum, 38–39
Angiography
  diagnosis of left main coronary artery disease, 27–36
  in pre-infarction angina in left main coronary artery disease, 21–22
Aorta
  acute dissection, 97–147
    introduction and medical therapy, 98–112
    medical therapy, 103–105
    panel discussion, 144–147
    results of medical therapy, 106
    surgery, 124–128
  ascending, cardiac anesthesia for lethal diseases of, 129–143
  in Marfan syndrome and other genetic disorders of connective tissue, 113–123
Artery
  great: *see* Transposition
  left main coronary
    anatomy, 2
    angiographic diagnosis, 27–36
    pre-infarction angina, 18–26
    severe stenosis, 2–17

Blalock-Hanlon procedure, 84
Bypass
  cardiopulmonary
    management after, 140–141
    termination, 139–140
  monitoring during, 139, 141

Connective tissue, genetic disorders of, aorta in, 113–123
Coronary disease, 1–52
  panel discussion, 49–52

Diagnosis
  angiographic, of left main coronary artery disease, 27–36

**Diagnosis,** *continued*
complete transposition of great arteries, 60–68
Dissection, acute aortic, 97–147
introduction and medical therapy, 98–112
medical therapy, 103–105
results, 106
panel discussion, 144–147
surgery, 124–128

Ehlers-Danlos syndrome, aorta in, 117–118

Halothane, 136
Heart rate, 132–133
Hemodynamics of pre-infarction angina in left main coronary artery disease, 20
Hemoglobin content, 133
Heparinization, 138
Herrick, J. B., 6–7
Hypothermia, deep, anesthesia for, 136–138

Induction of cardiac anesthesia, 134
Innovar, 135–136

Management, complete transposition of great arteries, 68–75
Marfan syndrome, aorta in, 113–123
Medications, presurgical, 129–130
Morphine, anesthesia with, 134–135
Mustard procedure, 85–87

Oxygen availability, myocardial, 131–132

Pathophysiology of complete transposition of great arteries, 55–60
Perfusion
flow rate and pressures, 138–139
heparinization, 138
management during, 138–139
monitoring, 139, 141
priming, 138
Premedication, 130–131
Priming, 138

Rashkind, 82–84

Septectomy, atrial, 84
Septostomy, balloon, 82–84
Stenosis of left main coronary artery, 2–17
clinical manifestations, 3–4
pathological manifestations, 3
surgical results, 4–5
**Surgery**
acute aortic dissection, 124–128
results in stenosis of left main coronary artery, 4–5
for transposition of great arteries, 77–91

Transposition, 53–95
complete, of great arteries
diagnosis, 60–68
management, 68–75
pathophysiology, 55–60
physiology, diagnosis, and medical management, 54–76
surgery, 77–91
panel discussion, 92–95
Treatment of pre-infarction angina in left main coronary artery disease, 22–23